# Teaching Ethics in Nursing

## A Handbook for Use of the Case-Study Approach

Minerva L. Applegate, EdD, RN
Nina M. Entrekin, MN, RN

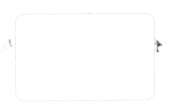

Pub. No. 41-1963

**National League for Nursing • New York**

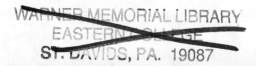

ISBN 0-88737-094-2

Manufactured in the United States of America

# Preface

In today's society, nurses are confronted with complex situations in clinical practice which demand ethical decision making and moral reasoning. The contemporary nursing curriculum must reflect the real world of nursing practice and prepare students to function in that world.

This handbook is written by and for and is addressed directly to nurse educators; it is an outcome of the authors' years of experience teaching ethics in health care to baccalaureate and master's nursing students. The handbook, which can be used in conjunction with a standard ethics or legal-ethical textbook, was designed to assist you in planning for your students learning experiences that will incorporate a variety of strategies for facilitating learning.

The purpose of this handbook is to offer you concrete suggestions for implementing one teaching method, the case-study approach. The selected strategies for implementation of the case-study approach have been used by the authors with nursing students either in selected classes or in a complete course focusing on ethics in health care. The case studies themselves are available in a separate format for student use; therefore your supplies can be replenished as needed. Resource lists are provided to serve as a vehicle for the further exploration of ethical problems and issues; while these lists are not exhaustive, they are intended to give direction.

We would like to acknowledge the input from many students, both graduate and undergraduate, at the University of South Florida College of Nursing who have shared their knowledge, values, experiences, and beliefs with us in the development of this content within the curriculm. We also appreciate the valuable input that we have had from our colleagues and peers during the development of this handbook. Finally, we would like to extend our appreciation to the National League for Nursing, for affording us the opportunity to share our ideas with other nurse educators.

# Contents

# 4.

# 1
# Ethics and Nursing

## INTRODUCTION

In a teaching session with fourth-year medical students, a physician from the United Kingdom was discussing American values as reflected in the American health care system. He said, "In England, people believe that they should be able to walk in the park without trumpets playing; in America, people believe that they should be able to play trumpets in the park."

To a nurse educator, this statement brought to mind several questions related to health care. In America, should we allow patients with terminal illness to die with dignity, in a calm, peaceful environment, or should we aggressively pursue every mechanism to maintain life, no matter what the cost or the stress patients and families endure? Should we quietly allow the congenitally handicapped to die, or should we do everything in our power to sustain life, no matter what the consequences for the individual, the family, or society? Should the patient be encouraged to be a passive recipient of care, or should the patient be encouraged to participate actively in the decision-making process? Should the nurse quietly sit back and observe the violation of a patient's rights, or should the nurse take a risk and become a client advocate? Should the nurse conform to institutional standards, or should the nurse maintain optimal standards at any cost? Should the nurse quietly assume a subservient role to other health team members, or should the nurse assert a positive and active role which supports her or his professionalism, no matter what the cost? Should the nurse always be supportive of colleagues and peers, or should the nurse support the patient even if it means challenging a colleague or peer?

The dichotomous situations in which a nurse frequently finds herself/himself may call for ethical decision making on a daily basis. How are nurses prepared for this decision making? In a time of unprecedented choices, how is the nurse able to differentiate between what is right and what is wrong? What does the nurse draw upon in order to resolve conficts with ethical overtones? Can ethical decision making be taught, and if so, *how* can it be taught?

The values prevalent in American health care seem to reflect a movement toward patients' rights, autonomy, freedom to choose, truthfulness, assertiveness, and shared responsibility and accountability. The movement in health care seems to be in the direction of trumpets blowing, and the quiet sitting on the park bench is frequently disturbed by the marching trumpeters.

As nurses, we have had a tendency in the past to stand quietly by, not making waves, assuming a posture of subservience, maintaining control in the patient situation, and letting other health care providers assume accountability for the outcomes of patient care, whether those outcomes were positive or negative. But our role has taken on new meaning as we move toward accountability, autonomy, and increasing independence in the patient-care situation. We can no longer afford not to become involved in the decision-making process as it relates to patient care. And as we become more assertive and more involved, we become more actively engaged in making decisions that impact upon patient care.

## THE SIGNIFICANCE OF ETHICAL DECISION MAKING IN NURSING PRACTICE

As nurse educators, we have a responsibility to prepare students for the real world of nursing practice. How do we prepare nurses for problem solving within the context of everyday nursing practice? How do we prepare students to make decisions when the situations they are presented with have ethical overtones, or when the nurse finds herself/himself in a situation demanding ethical decision making?

For example, what does the nurse do when caring for a young adult cancer patient who has chosen not to have any more treatments or tests performed? What does the nurse do when asked to witness a patient consent, knowing that the patient is not truly informed? What channels does the nurse go through if actions on the part of other health team members appear to have done harm to a patient? What does the nurse do when the physician tells the nurse to "no code" or "slow code" a patient, but the physician will not write the order on the patient's chart? Does the nurse tell the truth to a patient, when the patient has been given false information by other health team members? When told to discontinue life-support systems to a patient, to whom does the nurse turn for guidance and support? When told not to feed a newborn infant, how should the nurse respond? When observing signs of viability in a fetus that was intended to be aborted, what should the nurse do? When giving experimental drugs and not knowing the side effects or contraindications, what should the nurse do? When asked for information which other health team members did not give to the patient, should the nurse be truthful in responding? When ordered to violate a patient's autonomy and freedom, how should the nurse respond?

As the nursing profession has changed, its members have been confronted more and more frequently with situations demanding ethical problem resolution. The outcome of the resulting dilemmas has often been a feeling of ambivalence or of "aloneness," as reported in recent nursing studies.[1]

Nurses have been faced with unprecedented choices as a result of technological advances and new knowledge gained from the sciences. Life is prolonged with life-support systems and new treatments and therapeutic measures. While infants with multiple congenital anomalies are now given prolonged life, new questions of the quality of life are frequently presented to the decision maker in such situations. Patients are being exposed to many invasive procedures as a result of technological advances. Patients are demanding that choices and information be given to them.

Increasing government regulation has led to increasing consumer awareness. Health care providers have protested that their autonomy and independence are being threatened by external control measures that demand accountability in areas that in the past were traditionally controlled by the health care professions from within. Decision making has become more complex as the rules and regulations require increasing external review, peer review, involvement of other health team members, and involvement of families and clients in the decision-making process.

These issues are only a few examples of the real world of nursing practice, and they are not out of the ordinary. In reality, they are part of the nurse's everyday choices in clinical practice.

## THE USE OF
## AN ETHICAL DECISION-MAKING MODEL

A recent real-life episode illustrates a staff nurse's involvement in ethical decision making as part of her daily routine. The nurse's patient, Ms. B, age 39, was an intelligent, articulate professional woman with a diagnosis of terminal cancer. The patient, having experienced six months of continuous degeneration and repeated hospitalizations, expressed quietly to the nurse that she would refuse to have any more treatments or procedures related to the cancer. The patient stated that she "had been on a merry-go-round for the past six months, and it was time to stop." The patient was fully competent, not under sedation, and able to articulate her wishes clearly. She wanted to be involved fully in the decisions related to her care. The nurse offered to support the patient, informing her that she did have choices in terms of the decisions related to her care and that she should tell her physician that she wanted to be involved in the decision-making process. The outcome of

[1]Barbara L. Tate, *The Nurse's Dilemma: Ethical Considerations in Nursing Practice* (Geneva: International Council of Nurses, 1977). Minerva I. Applegate, "Moral Decisions in Selected Clinical Nursing Practice Situations." (Unpublished doctoral dissertation, Teachers College, Columbia University, 1981.)

the nurse-patient interaction was satisfactory to the patient. Following a physician-nurse conference and a physician-patient conference, with the patient's permission the nurse and the physician held a family conference for the purpose of clarifying expectations, exploring the family's knowledge of the patient's prognosis, and sharing the patient's wishes. The family noted that this was the first time that anyone had actually been truthful with them concerning the patient's prognosis. Decisions concerning the patient were, from that time until the patient's death, *shared* decisions, with input from the patient, the family, and members of the health team. The patient expressed satisfaction with maintaining some measure of control over her life, and the family were supported in the decision-making process.

How do we prepare nurses to engage in this type of ethical decision making? In situations like the one just described, how do we teach nurses to listen with all their senses to what the patient is saying? By communicating with the patient, the nurse must try to identify the ethical problem which has evolved in the patient-care situation. The roles of the various persons involved need to be clarified. The nurse must assess the situation and all of the intervening variables. The nurse needs to let the patient know that the nurse cares, and that the patient has a right to be involved in decisions related to his/her health care. Freedom and autonomy have to be promoted within the patient-care situation. The nurse needs to have enough autonomy and independence in decision making to be flexible and to consider alternatives and their possible outcomes. As a team member, the nurse has to be aware of other health team members' philosophies of patient care, and how those philosophies impact upon their decision making. Once the nurse has considered the alternatives, and predicted the outcomes of the alternatives, a choice must be made and the choice acted upon. Having acted, the nurse must compare the outcome of that action with her/his philosophy of patient care. Does the nurse feel comfortable with the outcomes of the decisions? Or should another alternative have been chosen? By these insights and with practice, the deliberative, rational process of ethical decision making can become more familiar and thus the basis for future decisions.

Ethical decision making within nursing practice served as a major component of the conceptual framework for this handbook. A systematic approach to ethical decision making was proposed by Murphy and Murphy in 1976; they suggested the following procedural steps: (1) problem identification, (2) ethical problem identification, (3) identification of the persons involved in the decisions, (4) identification of the role of the decision-maker, (5) consideration of the short- and long-term consequences of each alternative, (6) making the decision, (7) comparison of the decision with the decision-maker's philosophy of patient care ethics, and (8) a follow-up on the results of the decision in order to establish a baseline for making decisions in the future.[2]

---

[2]Mary A. Murphy and James Murphy, "Making Ethical Decisions—Systematically," Nursing '76 6:13-14, May 1976.

This approach is similar to Bergman's model for ethical decision making in complex situations.[3]

The model proposed by Murphy and Murphy was used as a guide for identifying situations in nursing practice that require moral decisions and for developing the case studies in this handbook. This model also assisted the authors in identifying the roles of the persons involved in various decision-making situations, as well as the types of decisions nurses were being required to make and their reactions to these situations. This type of model can be used by other nurse educators in teaching ethics to nursing students. It can also serve as a resource in the development and analysis of case studies. And finally, it can be introduced to the student as a means of analyzing case studies and, later, as a method for solving ethical problems encountered in professional practice.

For nurse educators, the process of ethical decision making is a teaching challenge. It promotes personal and professional growth in the educator as well as in students. Teaching ethics as applied to health care demands a constant exploration and awareness on the part of the educator. The educator will need to expand his or her theoretical base in areas such as philosophy, values, and the law. The close relationship between the legal and ethical parameters of professional nursing practice soon becomes evident. The educator must continually seek new information concerning contemporary issues having ethical overtones. New literature sources will be discovered by the educator, and the educator will discover that there is a very strong movement in health care based on the new field of study, bioethics. New relationships with faculty from other disciplines may develop. On almost any university campus, nurse educators will discover faculty from other disciplines who have explored bioethics and the application of philosophy to health care.

For example, the University of South Florida maintains a Division of Human Values within the College of Medicine. Appointed as affiliates within the division are faculty from a variety of disciplines, including even the president of the University. The disciplines represented include nursing, medicine, philosophy, religion, library science, communications, anthropology, social science, journalism, and psychology. As affiliate faculty, they participate in the planning, implementation, and evaluation of learning experiences which will foster in faculty and students an awareness of ethical issues and problems confronting health care providers. A monthly journal club meeting focusing on contemporary health care issues serves as an open forum for the discussion of issues. Initially, ten or twelve faculty attended the forums; after two years the division has outgrown its original physical space and attendance has grown to 35-40 faculty and students from a variety of disciplines, frequently including interested persons from outside the university. A human values newsletter is also now published four times a year, circulated to faculty and the public; it affords faculty an opportunity to present thought-provoking

---

[3]Rebecca Bergman. "Ethics—Concepts and Practice." *International Nursing Review* 20:140, November-December 1973.

articles related to ethical decision making in health care, as well as presenting information on local activities related to bioethics and upcoming opportunities for the development of knowledge and skills in this subject. After two years, the movement is encouraging faculty to become involved in ethical issues in health care from an interdisciplinary perspective. Although the initial commitment was to enhance the knowledge and skills of the affiliated faculty, the ultimate goal has been for faculty to integrate their new knowledge and skills into their respective teaching areas; this is fast becoming accomplished.

## TEACHING ETHICS IN HEALTH CARE

### Prerequisites for the Nurse Educator

Before you, the nurse educator, begin teaching a course in ethics to nursing students, there are certain suggested prerequisites that you should fulfill. One of the most important of these is the acquisition of a basic knowledge of moral philosophy and philosophical frameworks and of key philosophical concepts and terms. For example, you should be able to differentiate between *deontology* and *teleology,* in order to assist students in looking at the alternatives in ethical decision making. Basic terms and concepts such as *ethics, moral philosophy, moral institution, choice, reasoning, freedom, autonomy, rights,* and *values* have to be available as part of the educator's working knowledge and conceptual base.

You also need to explore contemporary ethical issues within the context of health care and consider the implications of these issues for health care providers. The only way to do this is to familiarize yourself with the contemporary literature related to bioethics and issues in health care. (See Chapter 4, Educational Resources.)

Another important prerequisite is searching out resource persons within and outside the educational setting who might assist you in the planning, implementation, and evaluation of course offerings. Is there a philosopher who is interested in ethics in health care, just waiting to be asked to participate in a new educational experience? Is there a physician who has participated in summer workshops in bioethics and wants to expand his involvement in this field? Is there a theologian who would be willing to assist you in broadening your background in moral philosophy?

One final prerequisite is that of taking advantage of educational opportunities for exploring ethics in health care. Be aware of seminars, workshops, discussion seminars, fellowships, and other creative opportunities that would enable you to explore health care issues with other interested professionals and experts in the application of ethics to health care.

In summary, before you undertake such a major task as developing an entire course in ethics as applied to health care, you should prepare yourself adequately, as you would for any other specialty area. Acquire the basic knowledge, go to the literature, seek out resource persons, and pursue learning experiences that will broaden your perspective and add to the depth of your knowledge base.

## The Case-Study Approach

What we are offering in this handbook are suggestions for one approach to teaching ethics, the use of the case study. As you read through the handbook, remember that all of the suggestions have been implemented by the authors in classroom situations, and that the outcomes with students have been positive. At the same time, we urge you to be flexible, and think about alternative ways in which you could best facilitate learning in your own students.

In our experience, the teaching of ethics in health care using the case-method approach has been most successful with senior nursing students, registered nurse students, and graduate nursing students. This is because, for the approach to be successful, the student needs to have had some exposure to the realities of clinical practice and at least a beginning comprehension of the ethical implications for health care providers. Our suggestions for student prerequisite learning will be explored in the next chapter.

Your personal philosophy, and your philosophy of nursing and health care will influence how you teach nursing students, and it may determine *what* you teach. As a nurse educator who teaches ethics, one positive outcome for you may be a gradual philosophical change within you. As you expand the body of your theoretical knowledge, you will discover in yourself a new capacity for making decisions within the context of health care. Other outcomes for you will be a new sense of accountability and an enhanced ability to engage in rational discourse with your colleagues and peers from many disciplines. Concepts such as *freedom, choice, values, autonomy,* and *accountability* will take on new meaning. You may even find that you, as a nurse educator, have opened new pathways for more creative thinking. At first, you may be uncomfortable with the fact that there are frequently many gray areas in decision making and that answers often do not fit neatly into black or white boxes. But let this frustration be motivating to you. The thing to keep in mind is that, as you grow, so will your capacity to engage in rational, deliberative, conscious decision making. This is the first step in a series of unexpected and pleasurable events that await you.

Now, let us explore the case-study approach for teaching ethics in nursing.

# 2
# The Case-Study Approach

The use of the case-study approach is not new to nursing education. The approach has traditionally been used to involve students in hypothetical situations prior to the application of concepts, principles, and skills in the clinical area. Clinical case studies often present patient care situations for which outcomes can readily be predicted. The outcomes of case studies involving ethical decision making are, however, less predictable, due to the complexity of human behavior.

The case study lends itself to learning experiences involving problem-solving objectives rather than to information and concept-learning objectives. The curriculum should provide the student with the prerequisite concepts and principles necessary in successfully solving problems, which ability is the core of nursing practice and underlies the role of the nurse as a professional.

As with any other teaching strategy, the case method has both advantages and disadvantages. Perhaps the major advantage is the reduction of patient risk. Students have the opportunity to practice decision making in *simulated* situations prior to their exposure to real-life decisions in *clinical* situations.

One disadvantage to using the case-study approach in ethics is that there is often no black or white answer to an ethical question. This confrontation with shades of gray may lead to frustration on the part of the learner as well as the nurse educator. Another disadvantage is the impossibility of making generalizations about outcomes because of the complexity and unpredictability of human behavior. At best, the nurse educator may only be able to foster in students an awareness of the existence of the ethical issues and problems that may confront them in clinical practice.

Gagne describes five categories of capabilities that humans learn; these are: verbal information, intellectual skills, cognitive strategies, motor skills, and attitudes.[1] The first three of these are hierarchical in nature. The teaching of ethics is complicated by the fact that the nurse educator is dealing with more than one type of human capability. Any ethical decision simultaneously involves information, intellectual skill, attitudes, and sometimes also cognitive strategy. *The goal for using the case-study approach in teaching ethics is to enable the student to go beyond the mere acquisition of information, concepts, and principles to actual problem solving and attitudinal change.*

As prerequisites to the case-study approach, the nursing curriculum should provide the student with the concepts and principles necessary to making ethical decisions. What prerequisite information should the student have? The authors suggest such things as:

—an introduction to terminology;

—an introduction to philosophical frameworks;

—a beginning knowledge of principles of ethical decision making;

—an awareness of the literature sources;

—an understanding of the roles of health team members;

—a knowledge of communications systems within the health care setting;

—an understanding of hospital policies and procedures;

—comprehension of the relationship between legal and ethical considerations of nursing practice; and

—an understanding of the relationship between accountability and autonomy.

A variety of techniques are available for presenting any given case study in a classroom or seminar setting. In selecting a specific technique, consideration should be given to the purposes and objectives of the learning experience as well as to situational realities such as group size and available resources. Presented in the following pages are: (1) a sample case study, followed by (2) an analysis of the case study, with (3) an identification of selected ethical issues, and (4) study questions that will assist the educator in facilitating classroom discussion of the issues and their implications for health care providers; these are followed by (5) a representative sample of eight suggested techniques for use of these materials.

## SAMPLE CASE STUDY:
### *INFANT WITH CONGENITAL ANOMALY*

Terry Smith, a three-week-old female infant, has been diagnosed as having non-communicating hydrocephalus. Gestational history revealed a normal pregancy and normal spontaneous vertex delivery following eight hours

---

[1] R.M. Gagne, *The Conditions of Learning* (3rd ed.) (New York: Holt, Rinehart and Winston, 1977).

of uncomplicated labor. The infant's birth weight was 7 lb., 6 oz. The only child of Jim and Mary Smith, Terry's birth had been anticipated with great expectations for the infant.

At the birth, the pediatrician noted that Terry's head circumference was greater than average, the scalp veins were distended, a tenseness and fullness of the fontanels was observed, and a widening of the cranial suture was evident. Severe spasticity in the legs was noted, and tendon reflexes were increased. The infant appeared lethargic, irritable, and had a sustained, high-pitched cry. Nuchal rigidity developed in the infant forty-eight hours after birth. A fever of undetermined origin developed and was present for two weeks. Physicians attempted to rule out meningitis. Nutritional failure of the infant was evident, and at three weeks of age her body weight was 4 lbs., 2 oz. Pneumoencephalography revealed the Dandy-Walker syndrome with cystic dilation of the fourth ventricle due to obstruction.

Following a team conference with the attending physician, the head nurse, the chief of staff of pediatrics, a neurologist, a surgeon, and a theologian, the physician met with the parents to discuss the infant's poor prognosis and to explore with the parents the possibility of performing a shunt. Terry's treatment at the time of the physician-parent conference had included intravenous fluids, formula by mouth, and antibiotics intravenously. Antipyretics had been ordered as needed, and anticonvulsants were to be given if the infant began convulsing.

Mr. and Mrs. Smith, after deliberating upon their decision for twenty-four hours, refused to sign a surgical consent for Terry to have a shunt procedure performed. They requested that extraordinary measures be discontinued and that Terry should be permitted to die a natural death. Antibiotics were to be discontinued, and the only nutritional sustenance to be offered was an I.V. of D/5/W to be run at 3-5 gtts./min. to keep the veins open for anticonvulsant medication if seizures should occur. The infant was to be N.P.O., but comfort measures were to be maintained. Ten days following the parents' decision, Terry expired. During that period of time the health care personnel were supportive to Mr. and Mrs. Smith, and opportunities were afforded the parents to express their feelings. They frequently visited the nursery, and both parents held the infant for long periods of time every day. When Terry expired, both parents stated that they were comfortable with their decision, and follow-up with the parents indicated that they both had worked through the grief process normally. Their future plans included having another child, and they appeared to be confident that their decision about Terry was mature and ethically justifiable in view of the high probability that Terry would not have been able to lead a full, productive, and normal life.

## ANALYSIS OF SAMPLE CASE STUDY

This case study presents several major ethical questions which relate to issues such as the quality of life, the rights of infants, euthanasia, parental rights, and health care provider rights. The role of the nurse in such a situation is complex. Both legal and ethical issues are of concern.

## Ethical Issues

The ethical issues involved in this sample case study would seem to be:

1. Withdrawal of life-support systems

2. Quality of life vs. sanctity of life

3. Infant rights vs. parental rights

4. Proxy consent

5. Health care provider rights, roles, and responsibilities

6. An exploration of alternatives within the situation

7. Guidelines for family support

8. Guidelines for the provision of comfort measures for the infant

9. An exploration of the personal support resources available to the nurse who is seeking support when caring for an infant who is being allowed to die.

## Study Questions

Study questions to which the efforts of group consideration might be directed, are:

1. When is it appropriate to withdraw support measures from a patient?

2. What are the legal constraints for the nurse who is ordered to withdraw life-sustaining support?

3. Should the nurse be involved in the decision-making process?

4. What type of support should the nurse offer the family?

5. How is it determined whose rights take precedence—the infant's or the parents'?

6. Does the nurse have the right to choose whether or not to participate in caring for an infant in a euthanasia situation?

7. From a philosophical perspective, how could one view this situation in a way that would present alternatives?

8. What is the role of the nurse as a health team member involved in a euthanasia situation?

9. How does one measure the quality of life?

10. To whom or what does the nurse refer for guidance and support when confronted with ethical issues and moral dilemmas?

## SUGGESTED TECHNIQUES FOR IMPLEMENTING THE SAMPLE CASE STUDY

Each of the following techniques for implementing case studies has been validated by the authors in the educational setting over a period of time. This is not presented as an exhaustive list, but merely as food for thought. The individual educator will undoubtedly discover new ways to implement the case-study approach, based on her/his experience and teaching situation.

### Small-Group Discussion

Small groups can be assigned any of a number of tasks or topics upon which to focus. Development of a *pro* or *con* position on an ethical issue delineated in the case-study analysis is one option. For the issue of infant rights vs. parental rights, for example, one group of students could be assigned the position that parents should always have the right to make decisions for their child; another group of students could take the position that the courts should make decisions for infants in cases where the decisions may not be consistent with societal norms. Have resources available to assist the groups in developing their position statements. Allow sufficient time for group interaction. Have each group designate a recorder who will be responsible for reporting the group's position on the issue. Lead class discussion for clarification and group consensus.

### Role-playing

Identify situations for role-playing from the case study. In this case, it could be the meeting between the physician and Mr. and Mrs. Smith to discuss Terry's prognosis and possible surgery, or it could be an interaction between the nursery nurse and the parents during one of their visits to their daughter. Delineate the role to be assumed by each volunteer or chosen participant. Assume one of the roles yourself if you feel it is appropriate. Have participants act out the roles they are assigned as they perceive the roles. Following the improvisation, lead a discussion of the role-playing to allow for analysis and reaction by the student observers. Seek group consensus on issues.

### Use of Audiovisuals

Select an audiovisual resource appropriate to the issues and theme of the case study. For this case, an appropriate choice would be the film "Who

Shall Survive?'', produced by the Kennedy Center for Bioethics. Have students identify situational factors common to the case study and the film. Promote further discussion for clarification and group consensus.

### Debate

Choose an issue or issues from the case-study analysis for the debate and identify brief *pro* and *con* position statements on each issue. The issue in the case of *Quality of Life* vs. *Sanctity of Life* might be indicated by the statements "A person's value may be determined by that person's ability to contribute to society" and "Every human being is considered sacred to God." Record the *pro* and *con* position statements on index cards. Distribute cards to students at random. Prenumber the cards in a logical sequence, alternating pro and con positions on the various statements. As you call out the numbers, the students read aloud their assigned statement and then justify their position. Promote group discussion of issues and positions with implications for health care providers.

### Panel of Experts

Select two or more individuals with varying perspectives on the central theme of the case study. For this case, consider a neonatologist, a "right to life" advocate, parents who have had the experience of a child with congenital anomalies, a theologian, a pediatric nurse, a philosopher, or an attorney. Distribute to the panel members, in advance of the class, materials that will assist in the discussion, such as a copy of the case study and its analysis. Introduce the speakers at the start of the class and summarize the case study. Moderate the panel. Following the panel presentations, encourage interaction between panel members and students for the purpose of clarification and consensus. This particular strategy lends itself to videotaping, and it is an ideal time for the educator to begin videotaping discussions on issues, which can be used in future classes. The authors, to date, have made two videotapes of such panel discussions, one on "The Allocation of Scarce Resources" and the other on "Truth Telling"; these have proved to be of great value in cost and convenience of repeating classes on these subjects. In addition, valuable discussions are not lost, but can be used to inform future groups of students.

### Study Questions

Provide students with copies of the case study and accompanying analysis, including the study questions. Distribute a selected bibliography on the ethical issues related to the case study. Assign each study question to a student, or, if group size dictates, to a team of students. Have the student or team explore literature related to the assigned question and report findings and answers to the question in class. Facilitate discussion of findings, clarify issues, and seek group consensus.

**Field Experiences**

Arrange field experiences relevant to the case study. For this case, consider arranging student visits to a center for the mentally retarded, an institutional review board meeting, a hospice, a day care center for the handicapped, a special education class, or a neonatal intensive care unit. Provide a copy of the objectives for the experience to the selected agencies and to the students. Have students sign up for one of the selected field experiences. Following the experience, have students write a brief summary of their reactions. Also have students report on their field visits in class. Lead group discussions to explore the impact of the first-hand observations upon students' beliefs or feelings about the case study.

**Student Presentations**

This technique is most appropriate for students with advanced standing. Present a variety of case studies from which each student may select the one in which she/he is interested. Provide copies of the case study, its analysis, and a list of essential readings for the topic to be presented. Serve as a resource to students as presentations are prepared. Provide guidelines for seminar discussion. Each student or group of students is responsible for discussion of the case study and relevant issues. Summarize and further explore the issue. Seek group consensus.

# 3
# Case Studies and Analyses

The case studies included in this handbook have been chosen to cover a wide variety of situations in which decisions were made by various actors in the situations—the patients, members of the health care team, the family. Various roles, various outcomes of decisions, and various patient care philosophies are depicted in the studies; these attempt to give the student the flavor of the clinical setting in which she/he may someday find it necessary to make difficult decisions ethically.

The case studies were developed on the basis of recent research findings, a review of the literature, and recent personal experiences of the authors; to the extent possible, they reflect the real world of nursing practice. Both of the authors have maintained their clinical practice; therefore, they are aware of the contemporary problems being encountered by nurses in the clinical setting and have incorporated this awareness into the situations presented.

## Using the Case Studies

Following each case study are the ethical issues suggested by the particular situation; these should be clarified through class discussion. Use of the accompanying study questions will help to clarify the issues; the questions will also assist students in determining the implications of the case study for nurses and other health care providers.

Using an ethical decision-making model, the educator should first assist the students in identifying the roles of the decision makers in the case study. The class should explore alternatives and identify the impact of the decisions on the participants in the situation, weighing the short-term and long-term consequences of each decision. Students should compare the outcomes of the decisions with their personal philosophies of patient care in order to assist them in making decisions in situations similar to the one under discussion.

Appropriate use of the case studies should foster in the students an awareness of contemporary issues with ethical overtones and should promote critical thinking in relation to the topics under discussion. Students should become aware of social, economic, cultural, and political variables that have an impact on health care. Students should become aware of the need to include members from other disciplines on the health care team when ethical problems arise that call for expanded expertise. Important concepts such as *freedom, justice, equality, autonomy, self-determination,* and *rights* should take on new meaning for the student engaged in the ethical decision-making process. The nurse-patient-physician relationship should begin to take on new dimensions, and the nurse's role as client advocate should be strengthened. Students should begin to incorporate principles of accountability and autonomy into their value system, and this should be reflected in their stated philosophy of nursing. The value they place on rational, logical thinking should also begin to increase, as reflected in the group discussions during seminars. The end result should be nurses who are at least minimally prepared to engage in logical, rational, ethical decision making in the challenging world of nursing practice.

The following twelve case studies and analyses were developed to assist nurse educators in the use of the case-study approach in teaching ethics in nursing. The case studies will be presented as follows:

Case Study  1: Terminal Illness

Case Study  2: Informed Consent

Case Study  3: Abortion

Case Study  4: Patient Abuse

Case Study  5: Patient Rights

Case Study  6: Brain Death

Case Study  7: Euthanasia

Case Study  8: Genetic Modification

Case Study  9: Captive Populations

Case Study 10: Allocation of Scarce Resources

Case Study 11: Human Experimentation

Case Study 12: Congenital Anomalies

## SYNTHESIS OF THE CASE-STUDY APPROACH

These case studies have been chosen to present a variety of simulated client situations that contain ethical considerations so that the student nurse may become aware of the process of ethical decision making within health care settings and to assist her/him in identifying the problems that may necessitate ethical decision making.

The case studies demonstrate that decisions may involve a variety of persons—health team members, the client, the parents, other family members, and perhaps community members such as theologians or other resource persons. Patients may be involved directly and cognitively in the decision-making process, as with the patient who was abused; in other situations, patient involvement may differ, as in the case of a fetus or a comatose patient.

The variety of simulated case studies also shows that the roles of decision makers vary, as evidenced in the difference between the physician who offered counseling and support to the family of the congenitally deformed child and the physician who rejected the family of the terminally ill adult client.

A discussion of the alternatives within each situation will promote in the student an awareness of the need to explore the effects which different actions will have upon the health care situation. For example, in the abortion case study, if the decision were made by the mother to have the child, the long-term effects upon the family could be phenomenal. These effects could be either positive or negative. The infant could become an integral part of the family structure, in spite of his or her handicaps, or the decision to save the infant's life could cast upon the family a tremendous economic, social, physical, and emotional burden. In the situation related to patient abuse, the short-term effects of the nurse's actions could promote temporary discomfort for the nurse in the immediate work environment, but the long-term effect could be improved patient care. The situation describing the terminally ill adult is another example of the consequences that may result when the decision maker chooses not to involve family in the decision-making process. The actual making of a decision and a comparison of the decision with the decision maker's philosophy of patient care ethics is also reflected in some of the case studies. For example, decisions were made at different times— either before action took place, during the event, or after the event; philosophies of patient care differ in the case studies, and evidence of a variety of role perceptions exists—counselor, advocate, protector, and in one situation, perhaps, the role of master.

The case studies also reflect the differences in outcomes of actions and decisions, an understanding of which may assist the student in making future decisions of an ethical nature. For example, in the situation of patient abuse, positive action by the nurse in spite of opposition led to change in the system, which would protect patients in the future. The situation with the terminally ill adult patient reflects the outcome of ethical decision making when family members or significant others are not included in the decision making.

## CASE STUDY 1:
### *TERMINAL ILLNESS*

Mrs. Sams, age 85, was admitted to the hospital one year after an extended radical mastectomy. Mrs. Sams had undergone a series of radiation treatments following surgery, and she was being treated with testosterone propionate for metastasis at the time of hospital admission, and the physician had informed the patient's husband and children that Mrs. Sams was not expected to live very long. The patient refused to take pain medication, and she was fully cognizant of the prognosis and aware of the rapidly deteriorating condition of her body. Mr. Sams accompanied his wife when she was admitted to the hospital. He also observed Mrs. Sams giving to the admitting nurse a sheet of paper on which she stated that she did want to be resuscitated if her heart should stop. Mrs. Sams was fully competent at the time of the admission, and she was not taking any medicine which would have affected her judgment.

Following admission to the hospital, during a three-month period of time, Mrs. Sams continued to deteriorate physically, but she was still alert and oriented. Her family visited her frequently, and, following a conference with the physician, demanded that Mrs. Sams be coded if she had a cardiac arrest. Mrs. Sams arrested three times and was coded. After the third time, the patient again wrote a note requesting that she not be coded, and she gave the note to the physician. The physician still would not write a "no code" order on the patient's chart. Finally, a nurse who had been caring for the patient since the time of admission did a "slow code' after a fourth arrest, and staff were unable to resuscitate the patient.

# ANALYSIS OF CASE STUDY 1

## Guidelines for Class Discussion

This case study presents several ethical questions that relate to issues such as: the quality of life; the rights and values of patients; family and health care providers; policies concerning the legality of the "living will"; hospital policies regarding "code" vs. "no code"; euthanasia, both active and passive; and legal considerations such as not following physicians' orders or the intentional act of delaying intervention which results in patient death.

## Ethical Issues

1. Code vs. No Code
2. Patient Rights vs. Family Rights
3. Death and Dying
4. The Living Will
5. Quality of Life
6. Euthanasia
7. Legal Considerations

## Study Questions

1. Should clear criteria be established for implementing a code/no code policy within hospital settings?
2. Should patients be consulted regarding the decision as to a code/no code order for the patient in case of a cardiac arrest?
3. Whose rights take priority in a code/no code situation—the patient's or the family's?
4. Should "living wills" be respected by health care providers?
5. Is a "no code" order an act of euthanasia?
6. Can health care providers be held legally responsible for not carrying out a physician's order to "code" a patient contrary to a patient's decision?
7. How does one measure the "quality of life"?

## CASE STUDY 2:
### *INFORMED CONSENT*

Mrs. Roy, age 70, was admitted to a hospital coronary care unit with unstable angina. Mrs. Roy's daughter was a nurse; she accompanied her mother to the hospital and visited her at least once daily following admission. Multiple diagnostic procedures were performed on the patient following admission. In the early hospitalization period, Mrs. Roy signed approximately fifteen consent forms for invasive procedures and triple-bypass heart surgery.

Although the patient was an intelligent, articulate individual, she was in a state of stress and anxiety about her hospitalization and impending surgery.

Each day, when her daughter came to the hospital to visit Mrs. Roy, she asked her about events during the day. According to the daughter, of the fifteen consent forms signed by her mother, few were truly informed and obtained in a non-stress state. When the daughter questioned her about the consent forms, the patient usually responded that she "had signed a paper for Doctor X because it was a test that he wanted to do."

Multiple complications resulted in a long convalescent period in the hospital. At the end of the two months, the patient's daughter estimated that in only three consent situations did the patient understand exactly what was being done to her, the risks and benefits of the procedure, and alternatives available to the patient.

## ANALYSIS OF CASE STUDY 2

**Guidelines for Class Discussion**

This case study presents several ethical questions for nurses which relate to issues such as: the conditions which must prevail if consent is to be truly informed; hospital policies concerning the procurement of informed consent; the nurse's role in protecting the patient in consent situations; and the patient's and family's rights relative to consent.

**Ethical Issues**

1. Informed Consent

2. Coercion

3. Patient Rights

4. Risk-Benefit Analysis

5. Patient Advocacy

6. Legal Considerations

**Study Questions**

1. What is meant by the concept of "patient rights"?

2. What are the criteria for a truly informed consent?

3. How can the health care provider assure that a patient is not coerced in a consent situation?

4. How extensive should a risk-benefit analysis be in a consent situation?

5. Does a patient have a right to refuse treatment?

6. What is the nurse's role in patient advocacy?

7. Can a nurse be held legally responsible if her/his assigned patient undergoes a procedure for which the consent was not fully informed?

8. What is meant by the terms "implied consent" and "proxy consent"?

9. How is consent obtained for a patient who is not mentally competent?

## CASE STUDY 3:
### *ABORTION*

Mrs. Allison, age 37, was a primipara in her fourth month of pregnancy. An intelligent career woman, Mrs. Allison and her husband had delayed having children until they had been married for ten years. Due to a family history of congenital anomalies and the patient's age, her physician recommended that amniocentesis be performed.

Mrs. Allison had the amniocentesis and returned to the physician's office for a prenatal checkup and to obtain the results of the amniocentesis. The physician informed Mrs. Allison that the fetus had Down's Syndrome. The physician and Mrs. Allison discussed options, and abortion was presented to the patient as one option for resolution of the problem. Encouraged to discuss the alternatives with her husband, Mrs. Allison stopped at the desk to speak to the office nurse. During their conversation, Mrs. Allison asked the nurse what she would do if she were in her situation. The nurse responded, "I cannot make that decision for you, but if I were in your situation, I would have an abortion."

## ANALYSIS OF CASE STUDY 3

**Guidelines for Class Discussion**

This case study presents several ethical questions which relate to the issues of abortion and amniocentesis, such as: the rights of the mother, of the father, and of the fetus; the use of amniocentesis as a screening mechanism; fetal experimentation; and the concept of values as an important component of ethical decision making.

**Ethical Issues:**

1. Right to Life vs. Right to Choose

2. Mental Retardation

3. Quality of Life vs. Sanctity of Life

4. Health Care Providers' Rights, Responsibilities, and Values

5. Fetal vs. Maternal Rights

6. Amniocentesis

**Study Questions**

1. Does the fetus have a "right to life"?

2. Does the mother have a "right to choose"?

3. Does mental retardation imply a diminished quality of life?

4. What are the basic premises underlying the "quality of life" versus "sanctity of life" argument?

5. Whose rights take precedence, the fetus's or the mother's?

6. Does amniocentesis present ethical issues to health care providers?

7. Does the health care provider have a right to express her/his own value judgments in a situation with ethical overtones?

8. Do health care providers have a right to choose whether or not to participate in a medical situation that causes moral conflict within the health care provider?

9. If a fetus is to be aborted, should fetal experimentation be permitted?

# CASE STUDY 4:
## *PATIENT ABUSE*

Mr. Winters, age 37, was returned to the medical floor following a chole-cystectomy. Routine orders for him included an intravenous solution of D/5/W to be infused at 30 gtts./min. for 24 hours. Fifteen hours after surgery, the nurse noted that the I.V. had infiltrated the patient's hand, and, following an unsuccessful attempt to restart the I.V., the nurse contacted the surgeon with a request that he restart the I.V. The surgeon was making rounds on the same unit that the patient was in, and he returned to Mr. Winters' bedside, examined the patient, and requested that the nurse bring him an intravenous set in order that he could restart the I.V.

Upon receiving the appropriate materials, the surgeon attempted six times, unsuccessfully, to restart the I.V. The patient complained of the pain and questioned the surgeon's competence. The surgeon became very angry, hostile, and abusive with the patient to the point of using profanity. The surgeon then left the patient's room and a resident was called to the floor and successfully restarted the I.V.

The nurse, having witnessed the interaction between the patient and the physician, remained with the patient, and who was visibly upset, allowed him to verbalize his feelings about the incident. Upon leaving the patient's bedside, the nurse immediately documented the incident fully on the patient's chart and conferred with the head nurse regarding the incident. The next day the nurse reported the physician incident to the chief of staff of surgery. The chief of staff met with the physician and informed him that his hospital privileges would be removed if any similar incidents were reported. The nurse was satisfied with the results of her actions and secure in the knowledge that nursing administrators had been supportive of those actions.

## ANALYSIS OF CASE STUDY 4

### Guidelines for Class Discussion

This case study presents many issues and concerns which have ethical and legal implications for the nurse, such as: patient rights; standards of care; client advocacy; protection of patients from harm; and the obligations and duties of health care personnel.

### Ethical Issues

1. Patient Rights

2. Client Advocacy

3. Concept of Harm—Physical, Emotional, or Social

4. Nurse-Patient-Physician Relationship

5. Responsibility and Accountability

6. Dignity of and Respect for Clients

7. Standards of Practice

### Study Questions

1. What are the ethical responsibilities of the nurse when a client's welfare is in jeopardy?

2. What actions should the nurse take to prevent potential harm to patients when the nurse judges another health care provider to be the agent of harm?

3. What are the nurse's legal responsibilities when a patient's welfare is threatened?

4. What channels are open to the nurse for communicating incidents of patient abuse and/or neglect?

5. What are the ethical considerations inherent within the nurse-patient-physician relationship?

6. How does the nurse demonstrate her respect for the dignity of patients?

7. What is the difference between responsibility and accountability?

## CASE STUDY 5:
### *PATIENT RIGHTS*

Mr. Mallette, age 62, was admitted to the hospital for repair of a fistula. While under general anesthesia, a biopsy of the prostate was performed on the patient. Following an uneventful recovery, the patient was discharged to home and instructed to return to the surgeon's office two weeks postoperatively for an examination. At the time of the office visit, the patient was discharged "in good health." Six months later, Mr. Mallette developed prostate symptoms and contacted a specialist for an examination. When he picked up his records to take to the consultant, the patient noted that the earlier pathology report of the prostate biopsy said "suspicious of adenocarcinoma." The patient had not been informed of the biopsy results by the attending surgeon at the time of discharge.

The patient informed his daughter, Ann, a nurse, of the biposy report. Consultation with the prostate specialist, after confirmation of the malignancy, resulted in treatment options of radical surgery or radiation for the cancer.

Mr. Mallette and his wife were given full disclosure by the consultant concerning the options and probabilities of treatment effectiveness. Their daughter, Ann, supported them in their decision making, and did not attempt to influence them in their decision. Ann also supported them in their personal decision not to charge the original surgeon with neglect, although Ann had very strong feelings concerning the original surgeon's lack of follow-up on the suspected carcinoma. At one point in the decision-making process, Ann's parents stated that it used to be easier when "physicians told you what to do... rather than having you make the choice." Committed to the patient's right to choose, Ann left the full responsibility of the decision making with her parents, believing that whatever they chose to do would be the best decision for them.

# ANALYSIS OF CASE STUDY

## Guidelines for Class Discussion

This case study presents a variety of ethical and legal considerations for the nurse, such as: the patient's right to be informed; health care provider neglect and malpractice; discharge planning needs for patients following biopsy procedures; accountability; and the nurse's role as a family member.

## Ethical Issues

1. Patient Neglect/Malpractice

2. Rights and Responsibilities of Health Care Providers

3. Truth-Telling

4. Discharge Planning and Accountability

5. Informed Consent

6. Incompetence

7. Conflict Resolution for the Nurse as a Family Member

## Study Questions

1. What are the rights/responsibilities of a nurse in a situation where neglect/incompetence has occurred?

2. What is the role of the nurse in discharge planning for clients who have had biopsy procedures?

3. In what health care situations, if any, should there be a question of truth-telling between patients and health care providers?

4. Do patients always desire the options for decision making in an informed consent situation for a life-threatening illness?

5. What responsibility do health care providers have to report other health care providers in neglect/incompetence situations?

6. How does a nurse resolve conflict and feelings of ambivalence when confronted with family situations evolving from neglect/incompetence on the part of other health care providers?

## CASE STUDY 6:
### *BRAIN DEATH*

Mr. and Mrs. James lived in a senior apartment complex. Mrs. James, age 80, was left alone at home while her husband went to the grocery store. Upon his return, Mr. James discovered Mrs. James on the floor of the apartment. She was not breathing, and had apparently experienced cardiac arrest. Mr. James called the emergency squad immediately. The emergency squad quickly transported Mrs. James to a nearby hospital, where the patient was admitted and immediately placed on a respirator. The patient remained unconscious, and at the end of the first month, evaluation revealed two flat electroencephalograms.

The physician met with Mr. James and his children to explore their feelings concerning Mrs. James's apparent brain death. The family could not comprehend brain death, and they pleaded with the physician to continue Mrs. James on the respirator.

The physician, after leaving the family conference, prepared to leave the hospital. On his way out of the unit, he verbally ordered a nurse to "pull the plug" on Mrs. James's respirator. The nurse, with the support of nursing administration, refused to "pull the plug." The physician was notified and returned to the hospital and himself discontinued the respirator. The physician then declared the patient legally dead. Staff offered appropriate support to the grieving family. The physician assumed full responsibility for his actions, and he did not criticize the nurse who had not followed his verbal orders.

# ANALYSIS OF CASE STUDY 6:

## Guidelines for Class Discussion

This case study presents a variety of legal and ethical considerations for the nurse, such as: the use of extraordinary measures for sustaining life; the determination of a patient's death; the rights of the patients, families, and health care providers when death is imminent; and acts of omission and commission on the part of the nurse.

## Ethical Issues

1. Quality of Life
2. Euthanasia
3. Extraordinary Means
4. Brain Death
5. Death with Dignity
6. Health Care Provider's Rights and Responsibilities
7. Legal Considerations: Omission and Commission of Orders

## Study Questions

1. What are the criteria for "brain death"?
2. When should health care providers institute life-support measures?
3. What are "extraordinary means" for sustaining life?
4. What are the rights and responsibilities of health care providers when caring for clients who can only be sustained on life-support equipment?
5. Under what conditions can life-support systems be withdrawn from patients?
6. What is meant by "death with dignity"?
7. Is removal of a life-support system considered to be euthanasia according to existing law?
8. What are the legal ramifications for health providers in situations demanding the institution or withdrawal of life-support equipment?
9. What is the role of the nurse in the development of standards for nursing personnel working with clients who are being maintained on life-support systems?

## CASE STUDY 7:
## EUTHANASIA

Mr. Haas, age 78, was admitted to the coronary care unit following an acute coronary occlusion due to a coronary thrombosis and atherosclerotic changes. The patient developed cardiac and respiratory arrest two days after admission and was placed on a respirator. It was determined that he was at level 5 consciousness: there was no reaction to painful stimuli; plantar, muscle, and tendon reflexes were absent; pupils were constricted and nonreactive to light; pharyngeal and corneal reflexes were absent; the patient was incontinent; and electroencephalogram readings were flat. One week following admission, the patient was removed from the respirator.

The family of Mr. Haas was frequently at the hospital, and a family member was always at his bedside during visiting hours. Mr. Haas had a son and a daughter who had been very devoted to him. His wife had died two years before, and he had been living alone and had been able to take care of himself without assistance from others prior to his hospitalization.

One month after Mr. Haas was removed from the respirator, his family requested a conference with the physician concerning his prognosis. The patient's condition was deteriorating, and the physician told the family that there was no hope that he would ever recover from his unconscious state. When family members requested a "mercy killing," the physician became angry and refused to discuss the situation any further. Family members continued to come to the hospital every day during visiting hours. They frequently spoke to members of the nursing staff concerning their wishes for a "mercy killing." The nurses ignored the family whenever they could, and little support was offered to them. Throughout this period the patient's condition continued to deteriorate, and the patient was resuscitated after several cardiac arrests. One year after the initial occlusion, the patient died.

# ANALYSIS OF CASE STUDY 7

## Guidelines for Class Discussion

This case study presents many questions of both an ethical and legal nature which have implications for nursing practice. Particular areas of concern relate to topics such as: "clinical death"; the use of extraordinary measures for life support; active and passive euthanasia; duties of health care providers; and family rights.

## Ethical Issues

1. Clinical Death
2. Extraordinary Measures
3. Death with Dignity
4. Euthanasia
5. Family Rights and Patient Rights
6. Health Team Members' Roles and Responsibilities with Dying Patients
7. Legal Considerations—Caring for Dying Patients

## Study Questions

1. Do criteria for "clinical death" ever vary according to the patient situation?

2. What is the nurse's role in the provision of family support when caring for terminally ill clients?

3. What criteria are used for determining when to institute or discontinue life-support systems?

4. What are "extraordinary" measures in relation to client care?

5. Is active or passive euthanasia ever ethically justified?

6. What are the client's and family's rights when a patient is dying?

7. What are the roles and responsibilities of the various members of the health care team who are providing care for the dying patient?

8. What are the nurse's legal responsibilities when caring for a dying patient?

## CASE STUDY 8:
### *GENETIC MODIFICATION*

Mrs. Lane, age 31, was admitted to the hospital with a diagnosis of metastatic carcinoma. Mrs. Lane had been hospitalized and treated one year earlier for carcinoma of the breast. At the time of the initial hospitalization, radical surgery had been performed, and the patient had been given chemotherapy and radiation. Mrs. Lane was married, and she had a two-year old child. Following the treatment for cancer, Mrs. Lane and her husband decided that they would like to have another baby, in spite of the fact that both had been warned of the possible teratogenic effects of Mrs. Lane's treatment for cancer.

When Mrs. Lane was admitted to the hospital the second time, for metastasis, she was five months pregnant. The metastasis was not treatable due to the pregnancy. During the hospitalization period, nursing staff were angry with the patient because of what they considered to be an irresponsible decision to become pregnant. Staff were unable to offer adequate support to the patient because of their judgmental attitudes.

Mrs. Lane remained hospitalized throughout the remainder of the pregnancy, and she delivered a viable infant. The patient died a few days after birth and the infant was transported to a major medical center via air ambulance due to methadone dependency at birth.

## ANALYSIS OF CASE STUDY 8

**Guidelines for Class Discussion**

This case study presents many ethical considerations for nurses, such as: value conflicts in patient care situations; fetal and parental rights; human experimentation; and the consideration of responsibilities to future generations and offspring.

**Ethical Issues**

1. Health Care Provider Values vs. Patient Values

2. Responsibility to Future Generations of Offspring

3. Human Experimentation

4. Genetic Manipulation Resulting from Treatment Modalities

5. Rights of Fetus vs. Rights of Parents

**Study Questions**

1. Do individuals have a moral responsibility to consider the quality of life for unborn generations?

2. How do health care providers' values make an impact upon the quality of care delivered to patients?

3. To what extent should health care providers respect the values of patients?

4. What are the responsibilities of health care providers and patients in situations which necessitate treatment with drugs that are known to produce genetic manipulation?

5. Does the fetus have rights?

6. How does the nurse resolve confict that evolves through differences in her/his own and the patient's value systems?

7. How rigorous is the consent process for human experimentation with treatments causing genetic manipulation that may affect future generations of offspring?

## CASE STUDY 9:
## *CAPTIVE POPULATIONS*

Joey, age 7, was committed to the children's psychiatric unit of a private hospital by his foster parents who were his legal guardians. Joey had been hospitalized in the past for psychiatric disorders, and he was under the constant treatment of a child psychiatrist. Joey's diagnosis was schizophrenia. He had been abandoned at the age of five, and his behavior had become increasingly abnormal since that time. Frequent acting out, hostility, violence, thought disorders, and hallucinations led to repeated hospitalization and a series of foster home placements. At the time of the current admission, he was under heavy sedation.

When Joey was admitted to the unit, Ms. Gomez was assigned to care for him. Standing orders on the unit were to restrain the children and place them in solitary confinement for two hours if they acted out or demonstrated behavior that was not controllable. Joey, as his sedation wore off, became hostile and angry with Ms. Gomez, screaming that no one loved him. Ms. Gomez, as ordered, restrained Joey and placed him in an empty, locked room for two hours so that he would "cool off" and not disrupt the unit. After several "cooling off" periods in solitary confinement over a period of several days, and with his condition worsened, Joey was transferred to a state mental hospital and permanently institutionalized.

## ANALYSIS OF CASE STUDY 9

**Guidelines for Class Discussion**

This case study presents many ethical and legal considerations for the nurse, such as: the rights of children; the consent process for captive populations; autonomy; and freedom.

**Ethical Issues**

1. Rights of Children

2. Rights of Captive Populations

3. Proxy Consent

4. Assault and Battery

5. Freedom and Autonomy

6. Standards of Care

**Study Questions**

1. When hospitalized for psychiatric conditions, do the rights of children differ from the rights of adults?

2. What is meant by the term "captive populations"?

3. What is the justification for "proxy consent" and under what conditions may it be legally challenged?

4. What constitutional rights are upheld when a patient is hospitalized for a psychiatric illness?

5. Under what conditions would the charge of "assault and battery" be upheld in a situation where a patient is hospitalized for a psychiatric condition?

6. What protective mechanisms are afforded the psychiatric patient to assure "freedom"?

7. What role does the nurse have in developing and implementing standards of care for the hospitalized psychiatric patient?

## CASE STUDY 10:
### *ALLOCATION OF SCARCE RESOURCES*

Susan Orr, age 6 months, was hospitalized for a congenital liver disorder. Susan was an only child, and her parents were devastated when physicians informed them that Susan would die within six months if a liver transplant were not performed. The parents, upon returning home with Susan, began to consider ways to procure a liver transplant for the child as soon as possible. In the upper-income strata, the parents spared no expense in the pursuit of a donor. Mr. Orr contacted the media and campaigned for a liver donor, using the child on television to promote sympathy among viewers. Mr. and Mrs. Orr mailed flyers to every hospital in the United States to plead for an available liver donor. Many hospitals posted the child's picture and the parents' plea in prominent view within the hospital emergency room.

Hospital staff in a small town posted the flyer with Susan's picture on it. Another family whose child was admitted to the emergency room after massive trauma saw the poster and requested that their child's liver be given to the child on the poster when the admitted child expired. The liver, following donation, was transported to a major medical center and transplanted in Susan. The transplant was successful, and the prognosis for Susan to lead a normal life was hopeful.

## ANALYSIS OF CASE STUDY 10

### Guidelines for Class Discussion

This case study poses many ethical and legal considerations for nurses, such as: the legal constraints of organ donation and transplantation; the use of the media for organ donor requests; justice in the allocation and distribution of scarce medical resources; and the rights of health care providers and consumers.

### Ethical Issues

1. Organ Procurement
2. Allocation of Scarce Resources
3. Use of Media to Promote Sympathy
4. Family Rights vs. Health Care Provider Rights and Responsibilities
5. Advertising for Organs

### Study Questions

1. What is meant by the term "allocation of scarce resources"?
2. Are there any conditions under which organs can be procured without the consent of the donor or the donor's next-of-kin?
3. In major transplants, such as heart and liver, what criteria for death are applied to the donor?
4. How are kidney transplants funded?
5. How are kidneys allocated from donor to recipient?
6. What are the responsibilities of health care providers in organ procurement?
7. What is the minimum age for giving permission for a kidney donation?
8. Should or should not the media be used as a vehicle for promoting sympathy for individuals in need of scarce organs?
9. Should or should not health care providers participate in promotion campaigns for the procurement of organs for individual recipients?

## CASE STUDY 11:
### *HUMAN EXPERIMENTATION*

Mrs. Adams, age 60, was hospitalized in an oncology center at a large metropolitan hospital. She was currently under treatment for metastatic cancer, and chemotherapy was being given on a daily basis. The drug being used for Mrs. Adams was approved by the Food and Drug Administration as a Phase II drug. A research protocol for human experimentation had been written by Mrs. Adams' physician and a copy of the protocol was on file in the oncology unit. The patient had signed a consent for treatment, and a copy of the consent was in the patient's chart.

Mrs. Casey, assigned as the primary nurse for Mrs. Adams, was ordered to give to Mrs. Adams a medication which was 100 times the recommended dosage of the drug. The nurse was unaware that the drug had been approved for a study, and the nurse expressed concern to other staff members about giving the drug. The nurse proceeded to give the drug as ordered, but she did not seek appropriate information sources as to its contraindications and side effects, although that information was available in the pharmacy and within the research protocol, which was available to attending personnel.

# ANALYSIS OF CASE STUDY 11

## Guidelines for Class Discussion

This case study presents a variety of ethical and legal considerations for the nurse, such as: roles and responsibilities of health care providers and patients within the context of human experimentation in health care; legal responsibilities associated with medications; consent; and health care providers' accountability.

## Ethical Issues

1. Human Experimentation
2. Informed Consent
3. Legal Responsibilities of the Nurse Related to Medications
4. Rights of the Terminally Ill Patient
5. Accountability

## Study Questions

1. How does one define "human experimentation"?
2. How are the subject and the researcher protected with informed consent in the human experimentation process?
3. What is a "research protocol"?
4. What criteria are used by the Food and Drug Administration to determine "phases" for drug experimentation?
5. Should or should not human experimentation be carried out with patients having terminal illness?
6. How does one protect a patient from "coercion" in the consent process?
7. What rights and responsibilities does the nurse have when assisting in the implementation of drug experimentation with terminally ill patients?
8. How does the nurse assure accountability when participating in drug experimentation studies?

## CASE STUDY 12:
### *CONGENITAL ANOMALIES*

George, a newborn, was born with multiple congenital anomalies. His parents, Mr. and Mrs. Smith, a young couple married one year, were totally unprepared to cope with the decisions which suddenly confronted them. The pediatrician conferred with the family and explained to them that the anomalies were both compatible and incompatible with life, and if George did have surgical repair immediately, he would probably be able to live, but would be severely retarded.

Mr. and Mrs. Smith, after conferring with the pediatrician, decided not to sign the consent for emergency surgery. In accordance with their wishes, the pediatrician immediately ordered withdrawal of all life-support measures for George, and an order was written for "comfort measures" only.

The pediatrician's orders were carried out by nursing staff for three and a half days. At the end of that period, the parents decided to have life-support measures reinstituted. Life was sustained, and the infant was transferred to a large medical center for immediate surgery. Following the surgery, the infant was sent to an institution for the remainder of his life.

## ANALYSIS OF CASE STUDY 12

**Guidelines for Class Discussion**

This case study presents many ethical and legal considerations, such as: who speaks for the child; euthanasia; extraordinary measures; and rights of infants, parents, and health care providers.

**Ethical Issues**

1. Quality of Life vs. Sanctity of Life
2. Proxy Consent
3. Extraordinary Means
4. Individual vs. Society
5. Family vs. Health Care Provider Rights and Responsibilities
6. Euthanasia

**Study Questions**

1. What is meant by the concept of "quality of life"?
2. What is meant by the concept of "sanctity of life"?
3. Under what conditions can "proxy consent" be legally challenged within the context of health care?
4. What would be considered "extraordinary means" for sustaining the life of a newborn infant with multiple anomalies?
5. What is meant by "comfort measures only" as applied to the newborn infant with multiple anomalies?
6. Is a nurse obligated to care for an infant when all life-sustaining measures have been discontinued, if the situtation causes severe moral conflict in the nurse due to the nurse's value system and philosophy of nursing?
7. Is withdrawal of all life-support systems from an infant with anomalies considered to be euthanasia from the legal perspective?
8. Should all life-support withdrawal situations be referred to an Ethical Review Board of multidisciplinary members who are prepared to engage in ethical decision making?

# 4
# Educational Resources

This chapter of the handbook is offered as a resource guide to the nurse educator who is interested in teaching ethics to nursing students.

The resources have been organized in the following categories: (1) teaching ethics, (2) ethical-legal issues, (3) general philosophy, (4) bioethics, (5) medical ethics, (6) professional ethics, (7) social ethics, (8) ethics and health policy, (9) environmental ethics, (10) reference sources, (11) journals, and (12) media resources.

Specific journal articles have not been included. The educator is referred to a recent National League for Nursing publication *Ethics in Nursing: An Annotated Bibliography,* (Pub. No. 20-1936) compiled by Terry Pence, Ph.D., for a comprehensive list of nursing ethics publications from 1901 to 1983. This book should be a required student textbook when teaching ethics in nursing; it will be referred to frequently in this section oas "Pence."

The resources presented in this chapter will assist the educator in acquiring a knowledge base and developing a framework for teaching ethics. The first section, *Teaching Ethics,* will introduce the educator to literature that describes the teaching of ethcis t.iat teaching ethcs in higher education. For specific readings in teaching ethics in nursing, see pp. 20-22.

Section 2 was developed to assist the educator in exploring legal and ethical issues from a broad multidisciplinary perspective. Pence has identified 34 topical issues that are of ethical concern to nurses. These issues correspond to the issues identified within the case studies in this handbook. Pence's annotated bibliography addresses specific nursing issues with ethical overtones. The educator, of necessity, must explore the literature outside s well as within nursing. Because of the multiplicity of issues confronting health care providers, the educator should not initially focus only on specific issues, but should acquire a feeling for the broad field of issues which may then be explored more specifically.

Section 3 refers the nurse educator to general philosophy books which cover a wide range of philosophical topics. The titles speak for themselves, and the reader is encouraged to peruse the list when seeking general background information for class discussion. In some situations, the educator may want to broaden her/his knowledge base, for example, in morality, theology, metaphysics, human values, rights, humanism, beneficence, equality, or ethical decision making. The list is not exhaustive, but the wide selection will give the educator some direction in terms of pursuing selected areas of interest. It will also assist the educator in indentifying contemporary authors who are publishing in the philsophical literature.

Section 4 refers the educator to selected readings in bioethics. The promotion of ethical decision making in health care has been stimulated as a result of inquiry in the field of bioethics. As stated by Bandman (1978), "..the function of bioethics is to explicate questions of moral rights" (p. xi) and the concern of bioethicists is that of exploring problems and issues in health care, identifying situations with ethical overtones, and applying principles of moral philosophy to assist health care providers in the resolution of problems encountered within the health care setting. The reader is again referred to Pence, particularly to the entry on "Books" (pp. 17-18) for an overview of nursing publications that would assist the educator in the conceptualization of bioethics as a relevant field of study for the exploration of ethical decision making in nursing.

Section 5 focuses specifically on medical ethics. Many of the readings have implications for nurses. It would behoove the nurse educator to become familiar with the medical ethics literature if the nurse educator is planning to use a multidisciplinary approach in the teaching of ethics to nursing students. For a contemporary overview of the nursing literature and the nurse-physician relationship, see "Doctor/Nurse/Patient Relationships: Models and Issues" in Pence (pp. 11-14).

Section 6 is designed to introduce the nurse educator to professional ethics from a multidisciplinary perspective which includes readings in business and law ethics. For the nurse educator interested in the historical evolution of professional ethics in nursing, see "History of Nursing Ethics: and "Ethics in Nursing Practice" in Pence (pp. 22-26).

Section 7 focuses on social ethics from a very broad multidisciplinary perspective. The impact of technology and its effects upon society and health care delivery will become a major discussion topic for the nurse educator teaching ethics in nursing. This list is far from exhaustive, but it will give direction to the nurse educator who is acquiring a knowledge base in bioethics.

Section 8 is closely related to section seven. The focus of this section is on public policy and its impact upon health care from a very broad multidisciplinary perspective. Contemporary topics include, for example: abortion; national health insurance; mental health policy; criminal jusice; allocation of scarce resources; population law; federal regulatory agencies; human experimentation; environment regulation; and genetics. Specific nursing literature references of interest will also be found in "Distributive Justice and Public Policy" in Pence (pp. 10-11).

Section 9 includes a brief list of readings in a selected area of content called environment ethics. These readings, although not extensive, were perceived to be important enough to categorize separately for the nurse educator who may develop a special interest in environmental ethics, or who may have a student interested in the environment.

Section 10 is a brief list of reference sources which will give direction to the nurse educator who is developing an expertise in teaching ethics in nursing. Of particular importance are the Literature Searches from the National Library of Medicine. The nurse educator interested in obtaining a current list of Literature Search titles should write to: Literature Search Program, Reference Section, National Library of Medicine, 8600 Rockville Pike, Bethesda, Maryland, 20209 (The educator should include her/his name and address typed on a gummed label, no return postage necessary).

Section 11 includes an alphabetized list of periodicals that frequently contain articles related to contemporary ethical-legal issues of import to health care providers. This list was developed following a careful perusal of current literature and the bibliographies of articles which focused on ethics in health care. It is not exhaustive, but it will give direction to the nurse educator who will be serving as a resource person for students who are exploring ethical issues in health care.

Section 12 is a list of media resources that will assist the nurse educator in acquiring learning resources such as audiovisual materials which may be used in the classroom to enhance student learning. At the present time, appropriate audiovisual resources are fairly limited in terms of availability for teaching ethics. The assumption is made that these resources will become more readily available as more nurse educators acquire an interest in and expertise in teaching ethics. Included in this list of selected resources are: 1) 16mm. films, 2) 35mm. filmstrips, 3) overhead transparencies, and 4) videocassettes. Also included is a brief list of sources from which educators may obtain information on educational media. The lists are not exhaustive, but they are intended to give direction to the nurse educator who is teaching ethics.

In summary, we are sharing with you our knowledge of educational resources that will assist you in the development of your knowledge and expertise as a nurse educator. This project has been a learning experience for us. Our reward will be—knowing that other nurse educators will be better prepared to assist nursing students in their movement toward enhanced ethical decision making in the health care setting.

## 1. Teaching Ethics

Barry, J.D., ed. *Ethics on a Catholic University Campus.* Chicago: Loyola University Press, 1980.

Bok, D. *Beyond the Ivory Tower: Social Responsibility of the Modern University.* Cambridge, MA Harvard University Press, 1982.

Callahan, D., and Bok, S., eds. *Ethics Teaching in Higher Education.* New York: Plenum Press, 1980.

Kohlberg, L. *Essays on Moral Development, Volume 1: The Philosophy of Moral Development.* San Francisco: Harper & Row Publishers, Inc., 1981.

Morrill, R.L. *Teaching Values in College.* San Francisco: Jossey-Bass, Inc., 1970.

Perry, W.G. *Forms of Intellectual and Ethical Development in the College Years: A Scheme.* New York: Holt, Rinehart and Winston, Inc., 1970.

Ruddick, W., ed. *Philosophers in Medical Centers.* New York: Society for Philosophy and Public Affairs, 1980.

Steele, S.M., and Harmon, V.M. *Values Clarification in Nursing.* New York: Appleton-Century-Crofts, 1979.

## 2. Ethical-Legal Issues

Aiken, W., and Lafollette, H., eds. *Whose Child? Children's Rights, Parental Authority and State Power.* Totowa, NJ: Rowman and Littlefield, 1980.

Annas, G.J., Glantz, L.H., and Katz, B.F. *Informed Consent to Human Experimentation: The Subject's Dilemma.* Cambridge, MA: Ballinger Publishing Co., 1977.

Applebaum, E.G., and Firestein, S.K. *A Genetic Counseling Casebook.* New York: Macmillan Publishing Co., Inc., The Free Press, 1983.

Arras, J., and Hunt, R. *Ethical Issues in Modern Medicine.* 2nd ed. Palo Alto: Mayfield Publishing Company, 1983.

Atkinson, G.M., and Moraczewski, A.S., eds. *Genetic Counseling: The Church and the Law.* St. Louis: Pope John XXIII Medical-Moral Research and Education Center, 1980.

Barnard, C. *Good Life/Good Death: A Doctor's Case for Euthanasia and Suicide.* Englewood Cliffs, NJ: Prentice-Hall, Inc., 1980.

Batchelor, E. Jr., ed. *Abortion: The Moral Issues.* New York: Pilgrim Press, 1982.

Batshaw, M.L., and Perret, V.M. *Children with Handicaps: A Medical Primer.* Baltimore: Paul H. Brookes Publishing Co., 1981.

Battin, M.P., and Mayo, D.J., eds. *Suicide: The Philosophical Issues.* New York: Pilgrim Press, 1980.

Bayles, M.D., and High, D.M., eds. *Medical Treatment of the Dying: Moral Issues.* Cambridge, MA: Schenkman Publishing Co., Inc., 1978.

Beauchamp, T.L., and Perlin, S., eds. *Ethical Issues in Death and Dying.* Englewood Cliffs, NJ: Prentice-Hall, Inc., 1978.

Beecher, H.K. *Research and the Individual.* Boston: Little, Brown and Company, 1970.

Beers, R.J., Jr., and Bassett, E.G., eds. *Recombinant Molecules: Impact on Science and Society.* New York: Raven Press, 1977.

Behnke, J.A., and Bok, S. *The Dilemmas of Euthanasia.* Garden City, NY: Anchor Press, 1975.

Benton, R.G. *Death and Dying: Principles and Practices in Patient Care.* New York: Van Nostrand Reinhold, 1978.

Bezold, C. *The Future of Pharmaceuticals: The Changing Environment for New Drugs.* New York: John Wiley & Sons, 1981.

Bluebond-Langner, M. *The Private Worlds of Dying Children.* Princeton, NJ: Princeton University Press, 1981.

Bier, W.C., ed. *Human Life: Problems of Birth, of Living, and of Dying.* New York: Fordham University Press, 1977.

Bok, S. *Lying: Moral Choice in Public and Private Life.* New York: Pantheon Books, 1978.

Boyd, K.M., ed. *The Ethics of Resource Allocation in Health Care.* Edinburgh: Edinburgh University Press, 1979.

Boyle, J.P. *The Sterilization Controversy: A New Crisis for the Catholic Hospital?* New York: Paulist Press, 1977.

Breggin, P.R. *Electroshock: Its Brain-disabling Effects.* New York: Springer Publishing Company, 1979.

Bulmer, M., ed. *Social Research Ethics.* London: Macmillan Press Ltd., 1982.

Burgdorf, R.L., ed. *The Legal Rights of Handicapped Persons: Cases, Materials, and Text.* Baltimore: Paul H. Brookes Publishing Co., 1980.

Burtchaell, J.T. *Rachel Weeping and Other Essays on Abortion.* Kansas City: Andrews and McMee, 1982.

Calibresi, G., and Bobbitt, P. *Tragic Choices: The Conflicts Society Confronts in the Allocation of Tragically Scarce Resources.* New York: W.W. Norton & Co., 1978.

Callahan, D., and Clark, P.B., eds. *Ethical Issues of Population Aid: Culture, Economics and International Assistance.* New York: Irvington Publishers, 1981.

Carson, R.N.; Reynolds, R.C.; and Moss, H.G., eds. *Patient Wishes and Physician Obligations.* Gainesville, FL: The University Presses of Florida, 1978.

Caughill, R.E., ed. *The Dying Patient: A Supportive Approach.* Boston: Little, Brown and Co., 1977.

Cohen, K.P. *Hospice: Prescription for Terminal Care.* Germantown, MD: Aspen Systems Corporation, 1979.

Chorover, S.L. *From Genesis to Genocide: The Meaning of Human Nature and the Power of Behavior Control.* Cambridge, MA: The MIT Press, 1979.

Cooke, R. *Improving on Nature: The Brave New World of Genetic Engineering.* New York: Quadrangle/The New York Times Book Co., Inc., 1978.

Corr, C.A., and Corr, D.M., eds. *Hospice Care: Principles and Practice.* New York: Springer Publishing Company, 1983.

Costhuizan, G.; Shapiro, H.; and Strauss, S. *Genetics and Society.* Cape Town, South Africa: Oxford University Press, 1980.

Curran, C.E. *Issues in Sexual and Medical Ethics.* Notre Dame, IN: University of Notre Dame Press, 1978.

Curran, W.J.; McGarry, A.L.; and Petty, C.S. *Modern Legal Medicine, Psychiatry, and Forensic Science.* Philadelphia: F.A. Davis Company, 1980.

Davis, J.W.; Hoffmaster, B.; and Shorten, S., eds. *Contemporary Issues in Biomedical Ethics.* Clifton, NJ: The Humana Press, Inc., 1978.

Devine, P.E. *The Ethics of Homicide.* Ithaca, NY: Cornell University Press, 1978.

Douders, A.E., and Peters, J.D., eds. *Legal and Ethical Aspects of Treating Critically and Terminally Ill Patients.* Ann Arbor, MI: AUPHA Press, University of Michigan, 1982.

Douders, A.E., and Swazey, J.P., eds. *Refusing Treatment in Mental Health Institutions—Values in Conflict.* Ann Arbor, MI: AUPHA Press, University of Michigan, 1982.

Durbin, P.T., ed. *Research in Philosophy and Technology, Volume 1.* Greenwich, CT: JAI Press, Inc., 1978.

Engelhardt, H.T., Jr., and Spicker, S.F., eds. *Mental Health: Philosophical Perspectives.* Boston: D. Reidel Publishing Co., 1978.

Ennis, B.J., and Emery, R.D. *The Rights of Mental Patients.* New York: Avon Books, 1978.

Erwin, D. *Behavior Therapy: Scientific, Philosophical, and Moral Foundations.* New York: Cambridge University Press, 1978.

Etzioni, F. *Genetic Fix.* New York: Macmillan Publishing Company, Inc., 1973.

Fersch, E.A. *Law, Psychology, and the Courts: Rethinking Treatment of the Young Disturbed.* Springfield, IL: Charles C. Thomas, Publisher, 1979.

Fields, F.R.J., and Horwitz, R.J., eds. *Psychology and Professional Practice: The Interface of Psychology and the Law.* Westport, CT: Quorum Books, 1982.

Finkel, N.J. *Therapy and Ethics: The Courtship of Law and Psychology.* New York: Grune & Stratton, 1980.

Fletcher, J.C. *Coping with Genetic Disorders: A Guide for Clergy and Parents.* San Francisco: Harper & Row Publishers, Inc., 1982.

_____.*The Ethics of Genetic Control: Ending Reproductive Roulette.* Garden City, NY: Anchor Press/Doubleday, 1974.

Fox, R.C., and Swazey, J.P. *The Courage to Fail: A Social View of Organ Transplants and Dialysis.* 2nd ed., revised. Chicago: The University of Chicago Press, 1978.

Freund, P.A., ed. *Experimentation with Human Subjects.* New York: George Braziller, Inc., 1970.

Friedman, P.R. *The Rights of Mentally Retarded Persons.* New York: Avon Books, 1976.

Furrow, B.R. *Malpractice in Psychotherapy.* Lexington, MA: Lexington Books, 1980.

Furstenberg, F.F.; Lincoln, R.; and Menken, J., eds. *Teenage Sexuality, Pregnancy and Childbearing.* Philadelphia: University of Pennsylvania Press, 1981.

Gallant, D.M., and Force, R., eds. *Legal and Ethical Issues in Human Research and Treatment: Psychopharmacologic Considerations.* New York: S P Medical and Scientific Books/Spectrum Publications, Inc., 1978.

Gaylin, W., and Macklin, R., eds. *Who Speaks for the Child: The Problems of Proxy Consent.* New York: Plenum Press, 1982.

George, J.E. *Law and Emergency Care.* St. Louis: The C.V. Mosby Company, 1980.

George, L.K., and Bearon, L.B. *Quality of Life in Older Persons.* New York: Human Sciences Press, 1980.

Glover, J. *Causing Death and Saving Lives.* New York: Penguin Books, 1977.

Goodman, R.M. *Genetic Disorders among the Jewish People.* Baltimore: Johns Hopkins University Press, 1979.

Grisez, G., and Boyle, J.M., Jr. *Life and Death with Liberty and Justice: A Contribution to the Euthanasia Debate.* Notre Dame, IN: University of Notre Dame Press, 1979.

Grobstein, C. *From Chance to Purpose: An Appraisal of External Human Fertilization.* Reading, MA: Addison-Wesley/Advanced Book Program, 1981.

Gutheil, T.B., and Appelbaum, P.S. *Clinical Handbook of Psychiatry and the Law.* New York: McGraw Hill Book Company, 1982.

Harzanyi, E., and Hutton, R. *Genetic Prophecy: Beyond the Double Helix.* New York: Rawson, Wade Publishers, Inc., 1981.

Hershey, N., and Miller, R.D. *Human Experimentation and the Law.* Germantown, MD: Aspen Systems Corporation, 1976.

Hilton, B.; Callahan, D.; Harris M.; and Condliffe, P. *Ethical Issues in Human Genetics: Genetic Counseling and the Use of Genetic Knowledge.* New York-London: Plenum Press, 1973.

Hofling, C.K., ed. *Law and Ethics in the Practice of Psychiatry.* New York: Brunner, Maxel, Inc., 1981.

Hoffman, J.C. *Ethical Confrontation in Counseling.* Chicago: The University of Chicago Press, 1979.

Holder, A.R. *Legal Issues in Pediatics and Adolescent Medicine.* New York: John Wiley & Sons, 1977.

Horan, D.J., and Delahoyde, M., eds. *Infanticide and the Handicapped Newborn.* Provo, UT: Bringham Young University Press, 1982.

Horan, D.J., and Mali, D., eds. *Death, Dying and Euthanasia.* Washington, DC: University Publications of America, Inc., 1977.

Houlgate, L.D. *The Child and the State: A Normative Theory of Juvenile Rights.* Baltimore, MD: Johns Hopkins University Press, 1980.

Hunt, R., and Arras, J. *Ethical Issues in Modern Medicine*. Palo Alto, CA: Mayfield Publishing Company, 1977.

Ingleby, D., ed. *Critical Psychiatry: The Politics of Mental Health*. New York: Pantheon Books, 1980.

Jackson, D.A., and Stitch, S.P., eds. *The Recombinant DNA Debate*. Englewood Cliffs, NJ: Prentice-Hall, Inc., 1979.

Kaback, M.M. *Genetic Issues in Pediatric and Obstetric Practice*. Chicago: Year Book, 1981.

Katz, J.; Capron, A.M.; and Glass, E.S. *Experimentation with Human Beings*. New York: Russell Sage Foundation, 1972.

Keane, N.P. *The Surrogate Mother*. New York: Everest House, 1981.

Kelly, P.T. *Dealing with Dilemma: A Manual for Genetic Counselors*. New York: Springer-Verlag, 1977.

Kieffer, G.H. *Bioethics: A Textbook of Issues*. Reading, MA: Addison-Wesley Publishing Company.

Kitcher, P. *Abusing Science: The Case against Ceationism*. Cambridge, MA: The MIT Press, 1982.

Kluge, E.W. *The Ethics of Deliberate Death*. Port Washington, NY: Kennikat Press Corp., 1981.

Kubler-Ross, E. *Death: The Final State of Growth*. Englewood Cliffs, NJ: Prentice-Hall, Inc., 1975.

Kuber-Ross, E. *On Death and Dying*. New York: Macmillan Publishing, Co., Inc., 1969.

Ladd, J., ed. *Ethical Issues Relating to Life and Death*. New York: Oxford University Press, 1979.

La Follette, M. *Quality in Science*. Cambridge, MA: The MIT Press, 1982.

Lakoff, S.A., ed. *Science and Ethical Responsibility*. Reading, MA: Addison-Wesley Publishing Company, 1980.

Lappe, M. *Genetic Politics: The Limits of Biological Control*. New York: Simon & Schuster, Inc., 1979.

Lasagna, L. *Life, Death and the Doctor*. New York: Alfred A. Knopf, 1968.

Law Reform Commission of Canada. *Sterilization: Implications for Mentally Retarded and Mentally Ill Persons*. Ottawa: Law Reform Commission of Canada, 1979.

Levy, N.B., ed. *Psychonephrology 1: Psychological Factors in Hemodialysis and Transplantation*. New York: Plenum Press, 1981.

Linacre Centre. *Euthanasia and Clinical Practice: Trends, Principles and Alternatives*. London: The Linacre Centre, 1982.

Macklin, R., and Gaylin, W., eds. *Mental Retardation and Sterilization: A Problem of Competency and Paternalism*. New York: Plenum Press, 1981.

Markle, G.E., and Peterson, J.C., eds. *Politics, Science, and Cancer: The Laetrile Phenomenon*. Boulder, CO: Westview Press, 1980.

Martocchio, B.C. *Living While Dying*. Bowie, MD: Robert J. Brady Co., 1982.

Masters, W.H.; Johnson, V.E.; and Kolodny, R.D., eds. *Ethical Issues in Sex Therapy and Research*. Boston: Little, Brown and Co., 1977.

McConnell, T.C. *Moral Issues in Health Care: An Introduction to Medical Ethics*. Monterey, CA: Wadsworth Health Sciences Division, 1982.

McLaren, A. *Birth Control in Nineteenth-Century England*. New York: Holmes & Meier, 1978.

Melton, G.V.; Koocher, G.P.; and Saks, M.J., eds. *Children's Competence to Consent*. New York: Plenum Press, 1983.

Miles, A. *The Mentally Ill in Contemporary Society*. New York: St. Martin's Press, 1981.

Miller, K.S. *The Criminal Justice and Mental Health System*. Cambridge, MA: Oelgeschlager, Gunn and Hain, 1980.

Milunsky, A., ed. *Genetic Disorders and the Fetus: Diagnosis, Prevention, and Treatment*. New York: Plenum Press, 1979.

Milunsky, A., and Annas, G.J., eds. *Genetics and the Law*. New York: Plenum Press, 1976.

Milunsky, A., and Annas, G.J., eds. *Genetics and the Law II*. New York: Plenum Press, 1980.

Moore, R.S., and Hormann, A.D., eds. *Consent and Confidentiality in Adolescent Health Care*. Arlington, VA: American Academy of Pediatrics, 1982.

Morris, R.K., and Fox, M.W., eds. *On the Fifth Day: Animal Rights and Human Ethics*. Washington, DC: Acropolis Books Ltd., 1978.

Munson, R. *Intervention and Reflection: Basic Issues in Medical Ethics*. Belmont, CA: Wadsworth Publishing Co., 1979.

Nevins, M.M., ed. *A Bioethical Perspective on Death and Dying: Summaries of the Literature.* Rockville, MD: Information Planning Associates, Inc., 1977.

Noonan, J.T., Jr. *A Private Choice: Abortion in America in the Seventies.* New York: Macmillan Publishing Co., Inc./The Free Press, 1979.

Noonan, J.T., ed. *The Morality of Abortion: Legal and Historical Perspectives.* Cambridge, MA: Harvard University Press, 1970.

Norwood, C. *At Highest Risk: Environmental Hazards to Young and Unborn Children.* New York: McGraw-Hill Book Company, 1980.

Office of Technology Assessment. *Genetic Technology: A New Frontier.* Boulder, CO: Westview Press, 1980.

Passmore, J. *Science and Its Critics.* New Brunswick, NJ: Rutgers University Press/Gross Lectureship Series, 1978.

Pattison, E.M. *The Experience of Dying.* Englewood Cliffs, NJ: Prentice-Hall, Inc., 1977.

Pope John Center. *The New Technologies of Birth and Death: Medical, Legal and Moral Dimensions.* St. Louis: Pope John Center, 1980.

Potts, M.; Diggory, P.; and Peel, J. *Abortion.* Cambridge: Cambridge University Press, 1977.

Ramsey, P. *Ethics at the Edges of Life: Medical and Legal Intersections.* New Haven: Yale University Press, 1978.

Ramsey, P. *The Ethics of Fetal Research.* New Haven: Yale University Press, 1975.

Reed, J. *From Private Vice to Public Virtue: The Birth Control Movement and American Society since 1830.* New York: Basic Books, 1978.

Regan, T. *All That Dwell Therein: Essays on Animal Rights and Environmental Ethics.* Berkeley: University of California Press, 1982.

Reilly, P. *Genetics, Law and Social Policy.* Cambridge, MA: Harvard University Press, 1977.

Riga, P.J. *Right to Die or Right to Live: Legal Aspects of Dying and Death.* Tarrytown, NY: Associated Faculty Press, Inc., 1981.

Rollin, B.E. *Animal Rights and Human Morality.* Buffalo: Prometheus Books, 1981.

Rosenbaum, M., ed. *Ethics and Values in Psychotherapy: A Guidebook.* New York: Macmillan Publishing Co., Inc./The Free Press, 1982.

Rosoff, A.J. *Informed Consent: A Guide for Health Care Providers.* Rockville, MD: Aspen Systems Corporation, 1981.

Rothstein, M.A. *Occupational Safety and Health Law.* St. Paul, MN: West Publishing Company, 1978.

Roy, D.J., ed. *Medical Wisdom and Ethics in the Treatment of Severely Defective Newborn and Young Children.* St. Albans, VT: Eden Press, Inc., 1978.

Russell, O.R. *Freedom to Die: Moral and Legal Aspects of Euthanasia.* New York: Dell Publishing Company, 1975.

Sass, L.B., ed. *Abortion: Freedom of Choice and the Right to Life.* New York: Facts on Life, 1978.

Schneider, C.E., and Vinovskis, M.D., eds. *The Law and Politics of Abortion.* Lexington, MA: D.C. Heath and Company, 1980.

Schrag, P. *Mind Control.* New York: Pantheon Books, 1978.

Segerstedt, T., ed. *Ethics for Science Policy.* Oxford: Pergamon Press, 1979.

Shuman, S.I. *Psychosurgery and the Medical Control of Violence: Autonomy Deviance.* Detroit: Wayne State University Press, 1977.

Sieber, J.E., ed. *The Ethics of Social Research.* New York: Springer-Verlag, 1982.

Simmons, R.G.; Klein, S.D.; and Simmons, R.L. *Gift of Life: The Social and Psychological Impact of Organ Transplantation.* New York: Wiley-Interscience, 1977.

Smith, D.E., ed. *Amphetamine Use, Misuse, and Abuse.* (Proceedings of the 1978 Amphetamine Conference.) Boston: G.K. Hall and Company, 1980.

Smith, W.L., and Kling, A., eds. *Issues in Brain/Behavior Control.* New York: Spectrum Publications, Inc., 1976.

Snowden, R., and Mitchell, G.D. *The Artificial Family: A Consideration of Artificial Insemination by Donor.* London: George Allen and Unwin, 1981.

Sorenson, J.R.; Swazey, J.P.; and Scotch, N.A. *Reproductive Pasts, Reproductive Futures: Genetic Counseling and Its Effectiveness.* New York: Alan R. Liss, 1982.

Stoddard, S. *The Hospice Movement: A Better Way of Caring for the Dying.* Briarcliff Manor, NY: Stein and Day Publishers, 1978.

Stone, A.A. *Mental Health and the Law: A System in Transition.* Rockville, MD: National Institute of Mental Health, 1975.

Sussman, A.N. *The Rights of Young People.* New York: Avon Books, 1977.

Swinyard, C.A., ed. *Decision Making and the Defective Newborn.* Springfield, IL: Charles C. Thomas, 1977.

Teichler-Zallan, D. and Clements, C.D., eds. *Science and Morality: New Directions in Bioethics.* Lexington, MA: Lexington Books, 1982.

Thomas, R.C., and Ruffner, J.A., eds. *Research Center Directory,* 7th ed. Detroit: Gale Research, 1982.

Tien, H.Y., ed. *Population Theory in China.* White Plains, NY: M.E. Sharpe, 1980.

Tietze, C. *Induced Abortion: A World Review, 1981.* 4th ed. New York: The Population Council, 1981.

Tsuang, M.T., and VanderMey, R. *Genes and the Mind: Inheritance of Mental Illness.* New York: Oxford University Press, 1980.

Valenstein, E.S., ed. *The Psychosurgery Debate: Scientific, Legal, and Ethical Perspectives.* San Francisco: W.H. Freeman, 1980.

Van Hoose, W.H., and Kottier, J.A. *Ethical and Legal Issues in Counseling and Psychotherapy.* San Francisco: Jossey-Bass, Inc., 1978.

Vardin, P.A., and Brody, I.N., eds. *Children's Rights: Contemporary Perspectives.* New York: Teachers College Press, Columbia University, 1979.

Varga, A.C. *The Main Issues in Bioethics.* New York: Paulist Press, 1980.

Veatch, R. *Death, Dying and the Biological Revolution.* New Haven: Yale University Press, 1976.

Wade, L.R., and Pritchard, M.S., eds. *Responsibility: Paternalism, Informed Consent and Euthanasia.* Clifton, NJ: The Humana Press, 1979.

Wall, T.F. *Medical Ethics: Basic Moral Issues.* Lanham, MD: University Press of America, 1980.

Walters, W., and Singer, P., eds. *Test-tube Babies.* New York: Oxford University Press, 1982.

Weir, R.F., ed *Ethical Issues in Death and Dying.* New York: Columbia Unversity Press, 1977.

Wilcox, S.G., and Sutton, M. *Understanding Death and Dying: An Interdisciplinary Approach.* 2nd ed. Sherman Oaks, CA: Alfred Publishing Co., 1981.

Wilson, J.P. *The Rights of Adolescents in the Mental Health System.* Lexington, MA: Lexington Books, 1978.

Winston, W.E., and Wilson, A.J.E., eds. *Ethical Considerations in Longterm Care*. Proceedings of a conference sponsored by Geriatric Research, Education and Clinical Center, Veterans Administration, Bay Pines, FL, and Eckerd College Gerontology Center, St. Petersburg, FL, 1977.

Wong, C.B., and Swazey, J.P. *Dilemmas of Dying: Policies and Procedures for Decision Not to Treat*. Boston: G.K. Hall, 1981.

Yelaja, S.A., ed. *Ethical Issues in Social Work*. Springfield, IL: Charles C. Thomas, 1982.

Zimring, F.E. *The Changing Legal World of Adolescence*. New York: Macmillan Publishing Co., Inc./The Free Press, 1982.

## 3. General Philosophy

Abernethy, V., ed. *Frontiers in Medical Ethics: Applications in a Medical Setting*. Cambridge, MA: Ballinger Publishing Co., 1980.

Abrams, N., and Buckner, M.D., eds. *Medical Ethics: A Clinical Textbook and References for the Health Care Professions*. Cambridge, MA: The MIT Press, 1983.

Annas, G.J. *The Rights of Hospital Patients*. New York: Avon Press, 1975.

Anna, G.J.; Glants, L.; Katz, B.F. *The Rights of Doctors, Nurses and Allied Health Professionals: A Health Law Primer*. Cambridge, MA: Ballinger Publishing Co., 1981.

Ashley, B.M., and O'Rourke, E.D. *Health Care Ethics: A Theological Analysis*. St. Louis: The Catholic Hospital Association, 1977.

Atiyah, P.S. *Promises, Morals and Law*. Oxford: Clarendon Press, 1981.

Barnette, H.H. *Exploring Medical Ethics*. Macon, GA: Mercer University Press, 1982.

Barrow, R. *Injustice, Inequality and Ethics: A Philosophical Introduction to Moral Problems*. Totowa, NJ: Barnes and Noble Books, 1982.

Barry, V. *Aspects of Health Care*. Belmont, CA: Wadsworth Publishing Co., 1982.

Basson, M.D., ed. *Ethics, Humanism, and Medicine*. New York: Alan R. Liss, 1980.

Beauchamp, T.L., and Childress, J.E. *Principles of Biomedical Ethics*. New York: Oxford University Press, 1979.

Bell, N.K., ed. *Who Decides? Conflicts of Rights in Health Care*. Clifton, NJ: The Humana Press, 1982.

Benditt, T.M. *Rights.* Totowa, NJ: Rowman and Littlefield, 1982.

Bliss, B.P., and Johnson, A.G. *Aims and Motives in Clinical Medicine: A Practical Approach to Medical Ethics.* London: Pitman Medical Publishing Co., Ltd., 1975.

Bloustein, E.J. *Individual and Group Privacy.* New Brunswick, NJ: Transaction Books, Inc., 1978.

Bodenheimer, E. *Philosophy of Responsibility.* Littleton, CO: Fred B. Tothman & Co., 1980.

Bondeson, W.B.; Engelhardt, H.T., Jr.; Spicker, S.F.; and White, J.M., Jr., eds. *New Knowledge in the Biomedical Sciences: Some Moral Implications of Its Acquisition, Possession, and Use.* Boston: D. Reidel Publishing Co., 1982.

Caplan, A.L.; Engelhardt, H.T., Jr.; and McCartney, J.J., eds. *Concepts of Health and Disease: Interdisciplinary Perspectives.* Reading, MA: Addison-Wesley Publishing Co. Advanced Book Program, 1981.

Carlton, W. *"In Our Professional Opinion . . . ": The Primacy of Clinical Judgment Over Moral Judgment.* Notre Dame, IN: University of Notre Dame Press, 1978.

Childress, J.F. *Priorities in Biomedical Ethics.* Philadelphia: Westminster Press, 1981.

Childress, J.F. *Who Should Decide? Paternalism in Health Care.* New York: Oxford University Press, 1982.

Christians, C.G.; Rotzoll, K.B.; and Fackler, M. *Media Ethics: Cases and Moral Reasoning.* New York: Longman, Inc., 1983.

Cohen, M., ed. *The Philosophy of John Stuart Mill: Ethical, Political and Religious.* New York: Random House, Inc., 1961.

Cohen, M.; Nagel, T.; and Scanlon, T., eds. *Medicine and Moral Philosophy.* Princeton, NJ: Princeton University Press, 1981.

Conrad, J.P. *Justice and Consequences.* Lexington, MA: Lexington Books, D.C. Heath and Co., 1981.

Curran, C.E. *Transition and Tradition in Moral Theology.* Notre Dame, IN: University of Notre Dame Press, 1979.

Dewey, R.E.; Gramlich, F.W.; and Loftsgordon, D., eds. *Problems of Ethics: A Book of Readings.* New York: The Macmillan Company, 1961.

Downie, R.S., and Telfer, E. *Caring and Curing: A Philosophy of Medicine and Social Work.* New York: Methuen, 1980.

Enhrenfeld, D.W. *The Arrogance of Humanism.* New York: Oxford University Press, 1978.

Englehardt, H.T., Jr., and Callahan, D., eds. *Knowing and Valuing: The Search for Common Roots.* Hastings-on Hudson, NY: The Hastings Center, Institute of Society, Ethics and the Life Sciences, 1980.

Feinberg, J. *Rights, Justice, and the Bounds of Liberty.* Princeton, NJ: Princeton University Press, 1980.

Fishkin, J. *The Limits of Obligation.* New Haven: Yale University Press, 1982.

Fletcher, J. *Moral Responsibility.* Philadelphia: The Westminister Press, 1967.

Fletcher, J. *Situation Ethics: The New Morality.* Philadelphia: Westminster Press, 1974.

Fishkin, J. *The Limits of Obligation.* New Haven: Yale University Press, 1982.

Fletcher, J. *Moral Responsibility.* Philadelphia: The Westminister Press, 1967.

Fletcher, J. *Situation Ethics: The New Morality.* Philadelphia: Westminster Press, 1974.

Fogel, D. and Hudson, J., eds. *Justice as Fairness: Perspectives on the Justice Model.* Cincinnati: Anderson, 1981.

French, P.A. *The Scope of Morality.* Minneapolis: University of Minnesota Press, 1979.

Gallagher, E.D., ed. *The Doctor-Patient Relationship in the Changing Health Scene.* Washington, DC: U.S. Government Printing Office, 1978 (Stock No. 017-040-00421-4).

Gaylin, W.; Glasser, I.; Marcus, S.; and Rothman, D. *Doing Good: The Limits of Benevolence.* New York: Pantheon Books, 1978.

Hannas, G.T.; Christian, W.P.; and Clark, H.D., eds. *Preservation of Client Rights: A Handbook for Practitioners Providing Therapeutic, Educational, and Rehabilitative Services.* New York: Macmillan Publishing Co., Inc./The Free Press, 1981.

Hare, R.M. *Moral Thinking: Its Levels, Method, and Point.* Oxford: Clarendon Press, 1981.

Hennelly, F., and Langan, J., eds. *Human Rights in the Americas: The Struggle for Consensus.* Washington, DC: Georgetown University Press, 1982.

Howard, T., and Refkin, J. *Who Should Play God?* New York: Dell Publishing Co., Inc., 1977.

Johnson, J., and Smith, D., eds. *Love and Society: Essays in the Ethics of Paul Ramsey.* Missoula, MT: American Academy of Religion, Scholars Press, University of Montana, 1974.

Kant, I. *Foundations of the Metaphysics of Morals.* Translated by Lewis White Beck, with Critical Essays. Ed. by Robert Paul Wolff. Indianapolis: The Bobbs-Merrill Co., 1969.

King, L.S. *Medical Thinking: A Historical Perspective.* Princeton: NJ: Princeton University Press, 1982.

Little, D., and Twiss, S.B. *Comparative Religious Ethics: A New Method.* New York: Harper & Row, Publishers, 1978.

Maestri, W.F. *Basic Ethics for the Health Care Professional.* Lanham, MD: University Press of America, 1982.

Marty, M.E., and Vaux, K.L., eds. *Health/Medicine and the Faith Traditions: An Inquiry into Religion and Medicine.* Philadelphia: Fortress Press, 1982.

McCormick, R.A. *Ambiguity in Moral Choice.* Milwaukee, WI: Marquette University Press, 1977.

McCormick, R.A. *Notes on Moral Theology.* Boston: University Press, 1981.

Mooney, G.H. *The Valuation of Human Life.* London: The Macmillan Press, Ltd., 1977.

Pavalon, E.I. *Human Rights and Health Care Law.* New York: American Journal of Nursing Co., 1980.

Regan, D.H. *Utilitarianism and Co-operation.* New York: Oxford University Press, 1980.

Rehr, H., ed. *Ethical Dilemmas in Health Care: A Professional Search for Solutions.* New York: Prodist, 1978.

Rogers, W.R., and Barnard, D., eds. *Nourishing the Humanistic in Medicine: Interactions with the Social Sciences.* Pittsburgh: University of Pittsburgh Press, 1979.

Rosenbaum, A.S. *The Philosophy of Human Rights: International Perspectives.* Westport, CT: Greenwood Press, 1980.

Shelp, E.E., ed. *Beneficence and Health Care.* Boston: D. Reidel Publishing Co., 1982.

Spicker, S.F., and Engelhardt, H.T., Jr., eds. *Philosophical Medical Ethics: Its Nature and Significance.* Boston: D. Reidel Publishing Co., 1977.

Mappes, T.A., and Zembaty, J.S. *Biomedical Ethics.* New York: McGraw Hill Book Company, 1981.

Preuss, J. *Biblical and Talmudic Medicine.* New York: Sandehrin Press, 1978.

Purtilo, R., and Cassel, C. *Ethical Dimensions in the Health Professions.* Philadelphia: W.B. Saunders, 1981.

Potter, V.R. *Bioethics: Bridge to the Future.* Englewood Cliffs, NJ: Prentice-Hall, Inc., 1971.

Rosner, F., and Bleich, J.D., eds. *Jewish Bioethics.* New York: Sanhedrin Press, 1979.

Shannon, T.A., ed. *Bioethics.* Rev. ed. New York: Paulist Press, 1981.

Shannon, T.A., and DiGiacomo, J.J. *An Introduction to Bioethics.* New York: Paulist Press, 1979.

## 5. Medical Ethics

Abrams, N., and Buckner, M.D. *Medical Ethics: A Clinical Textbook and References for Health Care Professions.* Cambridge, MA: The MIT Press, 1983.

Bliss, B.P., and Johnson, A.G. *Aims and Motives in Clincial Medicine: A Practical Approach to Medical Ethics.* London/New York: Pitman Medical Publishing Company, Ltd., 1975.

Brody, H. *Ethical Decisions in Medicine,* 2nd ed. Boston: Little, Brown and Company, 1981.

Burns, C.R., ed. *Legacies in Ethics and Medicine.* New York: Science History Publications, 1977.

Gorovitz, S.; Jameton, A.L.; Macklin, R.; O'Connor, J.M.; Perrin, E.V.; St. Clair, B.P.; and Sherwin, S., eds. *Moral Problems in Medicine.* Englewood Cliffs, NJ: Prentice-Hall, Inc., 1976.

Jonsen, A.R.; Siegler, M.; and Winslade, W.J. *Clinical Ethics: A Practical Approach to Ethical Decisions in Clinical Medicine.* New York: Macmillan Publishing Co., Inc., 1982.

McFadden, C.J. *Medical Ethics.* 2nd ed. Philadelphia: F.A. Davis Co., 1961.

McKinlay, J.B., ed. *Law and Ethics in Health Care.* Cambridge, MA: The MIT Press, 1982.

Pence, G.E. *Ethical Options in Medicine.* Oradell, NJ: Medical Economics Company, 1980.

Ramsey, P. *The Patient as Person: Explorations in Medical Ethics.* New Haven: Yale University Press, 1970.

Van Den Berg, J.H. *Medical Power and Medical Ethics.* New York: W.W. Norton & Company, Inc., 1978.

## 6. Professional Ethics

Atiyah, P.S. *Promises, Morals and Law.* Oxford: Clarendon Press, 1981.

Bayles, M.D. *Professional Ethics.* Belmont, CA: Wadsworth Publishing Co., 1981.

Begun, J.W. *Professionalism and the Public Interest: Price and Quality in Optometry.* Cambridge, MA: The MIT Press, 1981.

Behrman, J.N. *Discourses on Ethics and Business.* Cambridge, MA: Oelgeschlager, Gunn & Hain, 1981.

Bentham, J. *An Introduction to the Principles of Morals and Legislation.* Oxford: Clarendon Press, 1907.

Blair, R.D., and Robin, S., eds. *Regulating the Professions.* Lexington, MA: Lexington Books, D.C. Heath and Company, 1980.

Childress, J. *Moral Responsibility in Conflicts.* Baton Rouge, LA: Louisiana State University Press, 1982.

DeGeorge, R.T. *Business Ethics.* New York: Macmillan Publishing Co., Inc., 1982.

Dewey, J. *Theory of the Moral Life.* New York: Holt, Rinehart and Winston, 1960.

Engelbourg, S. *Power and Morality: American Business Ethics 1840-1914.* Westport, CT: Greenwood Press, 1980.

Frankena, W.K. *Ethics.* 2nd ed. Englewood Cliffs, NJ: Prentice-Hall, Inc., 1973.

Fried, C. *Contract as Promise: A Theory of Contractual Obligation.* Cambridge, MA: Harvard University Press, 1981.

Gerson, A., ed. *Lawyers' Ethics: Contemporary Dilemmas.* New Brunswick, NJ: Transaction Books, 1980.

Hoffman, W.M., and Wyly, T.J., eds. *The Work Ethic in Business.* Cambridge, MA: Oelgeschlager, Gunn & Hain, 1981.

Jonsen, A.R.; Siegler, M.; and Winslade, W.J. *Clinical Ethics.* New York: Macmillan Publishing Co., Inc., 1982.

Levine, A. *Free Enterprise and Jewish Law: Aspects of Jewish Business Ethics.* New York: Ktav Publishing House, 1980.

Sahakian, W.S. *Ethics: An Introduction to Theories and Problems.* Harper & Row Publishers, Inc., 1974.

Sherrer, C.W., and Sherrer, M.S. *Ethical and Professional Standards for Academic Psychologists and Counselors.* Springfield, IL: Charles C. Thomas, 1980.

Wolfman, B., and Holden, J.P. *Ethical Problems in Federal Tax Practice.* Charlottesville, VA: Michie/Bobbs-Merrill Co., 1982.

## 7. Social Ethics

Abelson, R., and Friquegnon, M. *Ethics for Modern Life.* 2nd ed. New York: St. Martin's Press, 1982.

Barbour, I.G. *Technology, Environment, and Human Values.* New York: Praeger, 1980.

Beauchamp, T.L. *Case Studies in Business, Society, and Ethics.* Englewood Cliffs, NJ: Prentice-Hall, Inc., 1983.

Durbin, P.T., ed. *A Guide to the Culture of Science, Technology, and Medicine.* New York: Macmillan Publishing Co., Inc./The Free Press, 1980.

Fisk, M. *Ethics and Society: A Marxist Interpretation of Value.* New York: New York University Press, 1980.

Fullinwider, R.K. *The Reverse Discrimination Controversy: A Moral and Legal Analysis.* Totowa, NJ: Rowan and Littlefield, 1980.

Godwin, G., ed. *Ethics and Nuclear Deterrence.* New York: St. Martin's Press, 1982.

Goodpaster, K.E., and Sayre, K.M. *Ethics and Problems of the 21st Century.* Notre Dame, IN: University of Notre Dame Press, 1979.

Hodges, L.W., ed. *Social Responsibility: Journalism, Law, Medicine.* Volume VII. Lexington, VA: Washington and Lee University, 1981.

Hoffman, W.M., and Moore, J.E., eds. *Ethics and the Management of Computer Technology.* Cambridge, MA: Oelgeschlager, Gunn and Hain, 1982.

Hohenemser, C., and Kasperson, J.X., eds. *Risk in the Technological Society.* Boulder, CO: Westview Press, 1982.

Institute of Medicine. *Health Care in the Context of Civil Rights.* Washington, DC: National Academy Press, 1981.

Kranzberg, M., ed. *Ethics in an Age of Pervasive Technology.* Boulder, CO: Westview Press, 1980.

MacIntyre, A. *After Virtue.* Notre Dame, IN: University of Notre Dame Press, 1981.

Monahan, J., ed. *Who Is the Client? The Ethics of Psychological Intervention in the Criminal Justice System.* Washington, DC: American Psychological Association, 1980.

Rappaport, D.C., and Alexander, T., eds. *The Morality of Terrorism: Religious and Secular Justifications.* New York: Pergamon Press, 1982.

Reamer, F.G. *Ethical Dilemmas in Social Service.* New York: Columbia University Press, 1982.

Rescher, N. *Unpopular Essays on Technological Progress.* Pittsburgh: University of Pittsburgh Press, 1980.

Ruse, M. *Darwinism Defended: A Guide to the Evolution Controversies.* Reading, MA: Addison-Wesley, Advanced Book Program, 1982.

Shinn, R.L. *Forced Options: Social Decision for the 21st Century.* New York: Harper and Row Publishers, Inc., 1982.

## 8. Ethics and Health Policy

Banta, H.D.; Behney, C.J.; and Willems, J.S. *Toward Rational Technology in Medicine: Considerations for Health Policies.* New York: Springer Publishing Company, 1982.

Bayer, R.; Feldman, S.; and Reich, W. *Ethical Issues in Mental Health Policy and Administration.* Rockville, MD: Alcohol, Drug Abuse, and Mental Health Administration, 1981.

Beauchamp, D.E. *Beyond Alcoholism: Alcohol and Public Health Policy.* Philadelphia: Temple University Press, 1980.

Beauchamp, T.C., and Pinkard, T., eds. *Ethics and Public Policy: An Introduction to Ethics.* Englewood Cliffs, NJ: Prentice-Hall, Inc., 1983.

Brody, B., and Beauchamp, T., eds. *Ethics and Public Policy.* Englewood Cliffs, NJ: Prentice-Hall, Inc., 1975.

Brody, B.A., and Engelhardt, H.T., Jr., eds. *Mental Illness: Law and Public Policy.* Boston: D. Reidel Publishing Co., 1980.

Brown, P.B., and Shue, H., eds. *Food Policy: The Responsibility of the United States in the Life and Death Choices.* New York: Macmillan Publishing Co., Inc., 1977.

Callahan, D., and Jennings, B., eds. *Ethics, the Social Sciences and Policy Analysis.* New York: Plenum Press, 1983.

Congressional Quarterly, Inc. *Congressional Quarterly's Federal Regulatory Directory: 1981-1982.* Washington, DC: Congressional Quarterly, Inc., 1981.

Ellston, F., and Bowie, N., eds. *Ethics: Public Policy and Criminal Justice.* Cambridge, MA: Oelgeschlager, Gunn & Hain, 1982.

Enos, D.D., and Sultan, P. *The Sociology of Health Care: Social, Economic and Political Perspectives.* New York: Praeger Publishers, 1977.

Feder, J; Holahan, J.; and Marmor, T., eds. *National Health Insurance: Conflicting Goals and Policy Choices.* Washington, DC: Urban Institute, 1980.

Finnin, W.M., Jr., and Smith, G.A. *The Morality of Scarcity: Limited Resources and Social Policy.* Baton Rouge, LA: Louisiana State University Press, 1979.

Fried, C. *Medical Experimentation: Personal Integrity and Social Policy.* New York: American Elsevier Publishing Co., Inc., 1974.

Ginzberg, E. *The Limits of Health Reform: The Search for Realism.* New York: Basic Books, 1977.

Grad, F. *The Public Health Law Manual.* Washington, DC: American Public Health Association, 1975.

Hannah, G.T.; Christian, W.P.; and Clark, H.B., eds. *Preservation of Client Rights: A Handbook for Practitioners Providing Therapeutic, Educational, and Rehabilitative Services.* New York: Macmillan Publishing Co., Inc./The Free Press, 1981.

Heidenheimer, A.J., and Elvander, N., eds. *The Shaping of the Swedish Health System.* New York: St. Martin's Press, 1980.

Hogue, L.L., ed. *Public Health and the Law: Issues and Trends.* Rockville, MD: Aspen Systems Corporation, 1980.

Hook, S. *Philosophy and Public Policy.* Carbondale, IL: Southern Illinois University Press, 1980.

Howie, J., ed. *Ethical Principles for Social Policy.* Carbondale, IL: Southern Illinois University Press, 1983.

Isaacs, S.L. *Population Law and Policy: Source Materials and Issues.* New York: The Human Sciences Press, 1981.

Jaffe, F.S.; Lindheim, B.L.; and Lee, P.R. *Abortion Politics: Private Morality and Public Policy.* New York: McGraw-Hill Book Company, 1981.

Krause, E.A. *Power and Illness: The Political Sociology of Health and Medical Care.* New York: American Elsevier Publishing Co., Inc., 1977.

Laslett, P., and Fishkin, J. *Philosophy, Politics and Society*. New Haven: Yale University Press, 1979.

Littlewood, R.N. *The Politics of Population Control*. Notre Dame, IN: University of Notre Dame Press, 1977.

Mappes, T.A., and Zembaty, J.S. *Social Ethics: Morality and Social Policy*. New York: McGraw-Hill Book Company, 1982.

Moore, M.H., and Gerstein, D.R., eds. *Alcohol and Public Policy: Beyond the Shadow of Prohibition*. Washington, DC: National Academy Press, 1981.

Pennock, J.R., and Chapman, J.W., eds. *Compromise in Ethics, Law, and Politics*. New York: New York University Press, 1979.

Poole, R.W., Jr., ed. *Instead of Regulation: Alternatives to Federal Regulatory Agencies*. Lexington, MA: D.C. Heath Company, 1982.

Regan, T., and Van DeVeer, D., eds. *And Justice for All: New Introductory Essays in Ethics and Public Policy*. Totowa, NJ: Rowman and Littlefield, 1982.

Rhoads, S.E., ed. *Valuing Life: Public Policy Dilemma*. Boulder, CO: Westview Press, 1980.

Richards, J., ed. *Recombinant DNA: Science, Ethics, and Politics*. New York: Harcourt Brace Jovanovich, Publishers/Academic Press, 1978.

Roemer, M.I. *Comparative National Policies on Health Care*. New York: Marcel Dekker, Inc., 1977.

Rothman, D.J., and Wheeler, S., eds. *Social History and Social Policy*. New York: Harcourt Brace Jovanovich, Publishers/Academic Press, 1981.

Somers, A.R., and Somers, H.M. *Health and Health Care: Policies in Perspective*. Germantown, MD: Aspen Systems Corp., 1977.

Swartzman, R.L., and Croke, K., eds. *Cost-Benefit Analysis in Environmental Regulation: Politics, Methods, and Ethics*. Washington, DC: Conservation Foundation, 1981.

Tancredi, L.R., and Slaby, A.E. *Ethical Policy in Mental Health Care*. New York: Prodist, 1977.

Thompson, F.J. *Health Policy and the Bureaucracy: Politics and Implementation*. Cambridge, MA: The MIT Press, 1981.

Veatch, R.M., and Branson, R., eds. *Ethics and Health Policy*. Cambridge, MA: Ballinger Publishing Company, 1976.

Weissman, G., ed. *The Biological Revolution: Applications of Cell Biology to Public Welfare*. New York: Plenum Press, 1979.

White, E., ed. *Sociobiology and Human Politics.* Lexington, MA: D.C. Heath and Company, 1981.

## 9. Environmental Ethics

Lexington, MA: D.C. Health and Company, 1981.

Partridge, E., ed. *Responsibilities to Future Generations: Environmental Ethics.* Buffalo: Prometheus Books, 1981.

Rodgers, W.H., Jr. *Handbook on Environmental Law.* St. Paul, MN: West Publishing Company, 1977.

Rogers, M. *Biohazard.* New York: Alfred A. Knopf, 1977.

Science Action Coalition and Fritsch, A.J. *Environmental Ethics: Choices for Concerned Citizens.* Garden City, NY: Doubleday Publishing Co./Anchor Press, 1980.

Shrader-Frechette, K.S. *Environmental Ethics.* Pacific Grove, CA: Boxwood Press, 1981.

Sills, D.J.; Wolf, C.P.; and Shelanski, V.B., eds. *Accident at Three Mile Island: The Human Dimensions.* Boulder, CO: Westview Press, 1982.

## 10. Reference Sources

Anglemyer, M.; Seagraves, E.; and LeMaistre, C., compilers. *A Search for Environmental Ethics: An Initial Bibliography.* Washington, DC: Smithsonian Insitution Press, 1980.

Bullough, B.; Bullough, V.; and Elcano, B., eds. *Nursing: A Historical Bibliography.* New York: Garland Publishing, Inc., 1981.

Cohen, M.L.; Stepan, J.; and Ronen, N. *Law and Science: A Selected Bibliography.* Cambridge, MA: Science, Technology and Human Values, Harvard University, 1978.

Goldstein, D.M. *Bioethics: A Guide to Information Sources.* Detroit: Gale Research Company, 1982.

Hastings Center, ed. *The Hastings Center's Bibliography of Ethics, Biomedicine, and Professional Responsibility.* Frederick, MD: University Publications of America, Inc., 1983.

Miller, A.J., and Acri, M.J. *Death: A Bibliographical Guide.* Metuchen, NJ: The Scarecrow Press, Inc., 1977.

National Library of Medicine: *Literature Searches.* Bethesda, MD:

> *Brain Death Criteria: January 1977 through April 1982.* 177 citations. Prepared by C. Kenton (No. 82-2).

*Human Experimentation: January 1973 through December 1975*. 291 citations. Prepared by C. Kenton (No. 76-4).

*Malpractice: January 1970 through April 1974*. 373 citations. Prepared by C. Kenton (No. 74-15).

*Malpractice in Hospitals, Dentistry, Nursing, Pharmacy, Veterinary Medicine and Allied Health Professions: May 1974 through September 1978*. 242 citations. Prepared by C. Kenton (No. 78-28).

*The Physician and Malpractice: May 1974 through September 1978*. 521 citations. Prepared by C. Kenton (No. 78-27).

*Transplantation: Ethical, Legal and Religious Aspects: January 1969 through January 1973*. 201 citations. Prepared by G.D. Nowak (No. 73-6).

Nevins, M.M., ed. *A Bioethical Perspective on Death and Dying: Summaries of the Literature*. Rockville, MD: Information Planning Associates, Inc., June 1977.

Pence, T. *Ethics in Nursing: An Annotated Bibliography*. New York: National League for Nursing, 1983.

Reich, W.T., ed. *Encyclopedia of Bioethics. Volumes 1-4*. New York: Macmillan Publishing Co., Inc./The Free Press, 1978.

Walters, L., ed. *Bibliography of Bioethics,* Volume 8. New York: Macmillan Publishing Co., Inc./The Free Press, 1982.

Wass, H. and Corrr, C.A., eds. *Helping Children Cope with Death: Guidelines and Resources*. Washington, DC: Hemisphere Publishing Corporation, 1982.

## 11. Journals

*Advances in Nursing Science*
*Allied Health*
*American College of Legal Medicine Newsletter*
*American Journal of Law and Medicine*
*American Journal of Nursing*
*American Journal of Psychiatry*
*American Journal of Public Health*
*American Medical News*
*American Psychologist*
*American Scientist*
*Annals of Internal Medicine*
*Behavioral Science*

*Bioethics Reporter: Ethical and Legal Issues in Medicine,
    Health Care Administration, and Human Experimentation*
*British Medical Journal*
*Bulletin of the American Academy of Psychiatry and the Law*
*Catholic Hospital*
*Canadian Nurse*
*Cancer Nursing*
*Citation*
*Congressional Quarterly Weekly*
*Ethics*
*Ethics in Science and Medicine*
*Federal Register*
*Hastings Center Report*
*Health Law Digest*
*Hospital Law*
*Hospital Progress*
*Hospitals*
*Human Life Review*
*Imprint*
*International Digest of Health Legislation*
*International Nursing Review*
*IRB (Hastings Center)*
*Issues in Health Care of Women*
*Issues in Mental Health*
*Journal of Advanced Nursing*
*Journal of Allied Health*
*Journal of Continuing Education in Nursing*
*Journal of Gerontological Nursing*
*Journal of Health and Human Behavior*
*Journal of Health Politics, Policy and Law*
*Journal of Legal Medicine*
*Journal of Maternal and Child Health*
*Journal of Medical Education*
*Journal of Medical Ethics*
*Journal of Medicine and Philosophy*
*Journal of Nurse Midwifery*
*Journal of Nursing Administration*
*Journal of Pediatrics*
*Journal of Psychosocial Nursing*

*Journal of Religious Ethics*
*Journal of Thanatology*
*Journal of American Association of Nurse Anesthetists*
*Journal of American College Health Association*
*Journal of the American Medical Association*
*Journal of School Health*
*Lancet*
*Law, Medicine and Health Care*
*Legal Aspects of Medical Practice*
*Linacre Quarterly*
*Man and Medicine*
*Medical Care*
*Medical Economics*
*Medical World News*
*Medico-Legal Bulletin*
*Medico-Legal Journal*
*Medicolegal News*
*Military Medicine*
*Modern Medicine*
*National Law Journal*
*Nephrology Nurse*
*New England Journal of Medicine*
*New Physician*
*New Scientist*
*Nurse Management*
*Nurse Practitioner*
*Nursing Administraton Quarterly*
*Nursing and Health Care*
*Nursing Law and Ethics*
*Nursing Leadership*
*Nursing Life*
*Pediatrics*
*Pediatric Annals*
*Pediatric Nursing*
*Perspectives in Biology and Medicine*
*Philosophy and Public Affairs*
*Philosophy East and West*
*Prism*
*Regan Reports on Nursing Law*
*Research in Nursin and Health Care*
*Review of Metaphysics*
*RN*
*Science*
*Science and Society*
*Scientific American*
*Social Biology*
*Stanford Law Review*
*Topics in Clinical Nursing*
*Western Journal of Nursing Research*
*WHO Chronicle*

## 12. Media Resources

In the listing that follows, the sources for 16mm films, for videocassettes, for 35m filmstrips, and for overhead transparencies are publication releases and the set of indexes produced by the National Information Center for Education Media (NICEM), University of Southern California, University Park, Los Angeles, CA 90007. These include: *Index to 16mm. Educational Films,* 7th ed., 1980; *Index to 35mm. Educational Filmstrips,* 7th ed., 1980; *Index to Educational Overhead Transparencies,* 6th ed., 1980; *Index to Educational Videotapes,* 5th ed., 1980; and *Index to Producers and Distributors,* 5th ed., 1980.

### *16mm Films*

"The Acceptance of Others — The Right to Die"

> *Time:* 30 minutes
> *Year:* 1971
> *Producer:* SREB
> *Distributor:* GPITVL

"Ethical-Legal Aspects of Nursing Practice"

> *Content:* death and dying, euthanasia, refusal of care, the living
> will, and family rights.
> *Time:* 30 minutes
> *Year:* 1974
> *Producer:* AJN
> *Distributor:* AJN

"Evolution by DNA—Changing the Blueprint for Life"

> *Time:* 22 minutes
> *Year:* not available
> *Producer:* DOCUA
> *Distributor:* DOCUA

"Moral Development"

> *Time:* 28 minutes
> Year: 1973
> *Producer:* CRMP
> *Distributor:* CRMP

"Should Man Play God?"

> *Content:* psychosurgery, fetal research, and abortions.
> *Time:* not available
> *Year:* 1973
> *Producer:* NBC
> *Distributor:* FI

"The Right to Life—Who Decides?"

> *Time:* 17 minutes
> *Year:* 1972
> *Producer:* LCDA
> *Distributor:* LCDA

"Who Should Survive?"

> *Content:* congenitally deformed infant, allowed to die.
> *Time:* 10 minutes
> *Year:* 1972
> *Producer:* KENJPF
> *Distributor:* KENJPF

### Videocassettes

"Are You Doing This for Me, Doctor, or Am I Doing It for You?"

> *Content:* medical ethics and human experimentation.
> *Time:* 52 minutes
> *Size:* ¾ inch
> *Year:* not available
> *Producer:* BBC (for NOVA)
> *Distributor:* T/L

"Nurse and Law Series: Rights of Patients, Part I; Rights of Patients, Part II."

> *Time:* 30 minutes
> *Size:* ¾ "
> *Year:* 1974 (Part I); 1977 (Part II)
> *Producer:* AJN
> *Distributor:* AJN

"The Gene Engineers"

> Contents: scientist's ability to transfer genes.
> *Time/Size:* 57 minutes/ ¾ "
> *Year:* 1977
> *Producer:* WGBH-TV (for NOVA)
> *Distributor:* T/L

"The Genetic Chance"

> *Content:* medical advances—amniocentesis; hemophilia.
> *Time/Size:* 57 minutes/ ¾ inch
> *Year:* 1978
> *Producer:* WGBH-TV (for NOVA)
> *Distributor:* WGBH-TV

"Ethics and Law in Nursing Practice"

> *Content:* problems, issues, and conflict in daily practice.
> *Year:* 1984
> *Time:* 60 minutes
> *Size:* ¾ " U-Matic, ½ " VHS, Beta I & II.
> *Available:* purchase or rental
> *Writer:* Leah Curtin
> *Distributor:* NMF

"Life or Death?"

> *Content:* ethical, medical, and legal issues surrounding "no code"
> and "slow code."
> *Year:* 1984
> *Time:* 25 minutes
> *Size:* not known
> *Available:* purchase or rental
> *Producer/Distributor:* NMF

### Videocassettes and 16mm Films

"Abortion Clinic"

> *Content:* "pro-choice" vs. "pro-life"
> *Writer:* Mark Obenhaus
> *Time:* 52 minutes
> *Year:* c. 1983
> *Producer:* PBS (for series, Frontline, hosted by Jessica Savitch)
> *Distributor:* FP
> *Availability:* color videocassette, ¾ ", ½ ", VHS or Betamax;
> purchase or rental.

"Code Gray: Ethical Dilemmas in Nursing"

> *Content:* congenitally deformed newborn; elderly-autonomy in
> nursing home terminally ill patient allocation of scarce
> resources.
> *Writers:* Ben Achtenberg and Joan Sawyer in collaboration with
> Christine Miller.

*Time:* 28 minutes
*Year:* c. 1983
*Producer:* BOS
*Distributor:* FP
*Availability:* ½", color videocassette, ¾", VHS or Betamax
  purchase. Color film, 16mm., purchase or rental.

"Ethics, Law and Nursing: Dealing with Problems, Issues and Conflict in Daily Practice"

  *Content:* vignettes depicting hospital nursing situations followed by
    discussion.
  *Writer:* Leah L. Curtin
  *Format:* three units, study guides, and bibliography
  *Time:* 60 minutes
  *Year:* c. 1983
  *Producer:* Leah L. Curtin
  *Distributor:* NMF
  *Availability:* videocassette, ¾", ½" Beta I, Beta II—purchase. Six
    minute overview available for preview.

"Trying Times: Crisis in Fertility"

  *Content:* alternatives—including adoption and artificial insemi-
    nation.
  *Writer:* Joan Sawyer in collaboration with Barbara Eck Menning
  *Time:* 33 minutes
  *Year:* c. 1983
  *Producer:* Sawyer/Menning
  *Distributor:* FP
  *Availability:* color videocassette, ¾", ½", VHS or Betamax—pur-
    chase. Color film, 16mm., purchase or rental.

## Overhead Transparencies

"Ethical and Moral Development"

  *Size:* 8" x 10"
  *Number of Transparencies:* 16
  *Year:* 1975
  *Producer/Distributor:* LANSFD

"Facing Issues of Life and Death"

> *Content:* euthanasia, transplants, abortion, genetic experimenta
> tion, informed consent, brain research, and quality of
> medical care.
> *Size:* 10 " x 10 "
> *Number of Transparencies:* 12
> *Producer/Distributor:* MILKEN

"Bill of Rights"

> *Content:* basic human rights in democracy: speech, privacy, and
> religion.
> *Size:* 8 " x 10 "
> *Number of Transparencies:* 13
> *Producer/Distributor:* AEVAC

### 35mm. Filmstrips

"Ethics and the Hospital"

> *Content:* hospital ethics, patient privacy, and safety
> *Number of Frames:* 131
> *Year:* 1971
> *Format:* sound filmstrip/audiotape
> *Producer/Distributor:* TRNAID

"The Holocaust, Part I—Without Pity"

> *Content:* personal experiences, degradation, dehumanization
> *Number of Frames:* 69
> *Year:* 1977
> *Format:* filmstrip with record, cassette, and script
> *Producer/Distributor:* AVNA

"The Holocaust, Part II—Dream Into Reality"

> *Content:* historical and political perspectives
> *Number of Frames:* 74
> *Year:* 1977
> *Format:* filmstrip with record, cassette, and script
> *Producer/Distributor:* AVNA

"Human Rights—Who Speaks for Man?"

> *Content:* international perspective on human rights
> *Number of Frames:* 74
> *Year:* 1978
> *Format:* filmstrip with cassette and script
> *Producer/Distributor:* CAF

## Coding for Producers/Distributors

AEVAC      Aevac, Inc.
1500 Park Avenue
South Plainfield, NJ 07080

AJN      American Journal of Nursing
555 W. 57th Street
New York, NY 10019

AVNA      Audiovisual Narrative Arts
P.O. Box 9
Pleasantville, NY 10570

BBC      British Broadcasting Corporation, TV
30 Fifth Avenue
New York, NY 10020

BOS      Boston Film/Video Foundation
The Foundation for Visual Communication
25 Church Street
Boston MA 02116

CAF      Current Affairs Films, Div. of Key Products
24 Danbury Road
Wilton, CT 06897

CRMP      CRM Education Films
Del Mar, CA 92014

FI      Films Incorporated
733 Green Bay Road
Wilmette, IL 60091

FP      Film Pharos, Inc.
701 W. Willow Street
Chicago, IL 60604

GPITVL      Great Plains Instructional TV Library
University of Nebraska
P.O. Box 80669
Lincoln NE 68505

INT      Interaction Inc.
680 N. 74th Street
Wauwatosa, WI 53213

| | |
|---|---|
| KENJPF | Joseph P. Kennedy, Jr. Foundation<br>1701 K Street, N.W.<br>Washington, DC 20006 |
| LANSFD | Lansford Publishing Company<br>P.O. Box 8711<br>1088 Lincoln Avenue<br>San Jose, CA 95155 |
| LCOA | Learning Corporation of America<br>1350 Avenue of Americas<br>New York, NY 10019 |
| MILKEN | Milliken Publishing Company<br>611 Olive Street<br>St. Louis, MO 63101 |
| NBC | National Broadcasting Company, Inc.<br>30 Rockefeller Plaza<br>New York, NY 10020 |
| NMF | Nursing Management Films<br>600 South Federal Street<br>Chicago, IL 60605 |
| NOVA | Nova Studios<br>145 E. 49th Street<br>New York, NY 10017 |
| PBS | Public Broadcasting Service<br>475 L'Enfant Plaza, S.W.<br>Washington, DC 20024 |
| SREB | Southern Regional Educational Board<br>130 Sixth Street, N.W.<br>Atlanta, GA 30313 |
| TL | Teachers Library, Inc.<br>15 Columbus Circle<br>New York, NY 10023 |
| TRNAID | Train-Aide Educational Systems<br>1015 Grandview<br>Glendale, CA 91201 |
| WGBH | WGBH<br>125 Western Avenue<br>Boston, MA 02134 |

**Other Sources for Obtaining
Information on Education Media**

American Film Review: Films of America
    Publisher: The American Education and Historical Film Center
        St. Davids, PA 19087

Documents of International Organizations: A Bibliographic Handbook
    Publisher: American Library Association
        50 East Huron Street
        Chicago, IL 60611

Educators' Guide to Free Films
    Publisher: Educators' Progress Service, Inc.
        Randolph, WI 53956

Educators' Guide to Free Filmstrips
    Publisher: Educators' Progress Service, Inc.
        Randolph, WI 53956

Educators' Guide to Free Tapes, Scripts, and Transcripts
    Publisher: Educators' Progress Service, Inc.
        Randolph, WI 53956

ERIC Clearinghouse on Educational Media and Technology
    Publisher: ERIC Clearinghouse
        Box E, School of Education
        Stanford University
        Stanford, CA 94305

Film Reference Guide for Medicine and Allied Sciences
    Publisher: Superintendent of Documents
        U.S. Government Printing Office
        Washington, DC 10402

Index to Instructional Media Catalogs
    Publisher: R.R. Bowker Company
        1180 Avenue of the Americas
        New York, NY 10036

# About the Authors

**Dr. Minerva Applegate** is an associate professor at the University of South Florida College of Nursing, Tampa. She is also an affiliate associate professor in the Division of Human Values, Department of Comprehensive Medicine, and a faculty member in the Department of Family Medicine at the University of South Florida College of Medicine.

At the present time, Dr. Applegate, in addition to teaching ethics in health care, is also serving as Project Director for a Kellogg Foundation Grant to prepare community college teachers at the graduate level. She is employed part-time as a staff nurse in rehabilitation at Bayfront Medical Center, St. Petersburg.

Dr. Applegate was awarded an Associate in Applied Science in Nursing from Ocean County College, New Jersey, a Bachelor of Science in Nursing from the University of Miami, Florida, and a Master of Education and Doctor of Education from Teachers College, Columbia University. She completed courses in bioethics at Georgetown University, Kennedy Center for Bioethics, and she recently returned to Teachers College, Columbia University, to do post-doctoral study in educational administration.

Dr. Applegate serves on the Editorial Advisory Board for *Nurse Educator,* and she is presently coordinating a multidisciplinary publication project in medical education.

**Nina M. Entrekin** is an associate professor at the University of South Florida College of Nursing, Tampa, where she is Director of the Instructional Materials Center in addition to her teaching responsibilities. She is a nurse clinician in the University of South Florida Medical Center's comprehensive breast cancer diagnosis and treatment program.

Ms. Entrekin received her Bachelor of Science in Nursing and Master in Nursing degrees from Emory University in Atlanta, Georgia. She is a candidate for the Ph.D. degree at Florida State University in the area of Instructional Design and Development.

Ms. Entrekin is an active volunteer with the Florida Division of the American Cancer Society, serving on the Nursing Committee and coordinating and presenting continuing education programs for oncology nurses. She is a consultant in mediated instructional systems and establishing learning resource centers and is listed in *Who's Who in American Nursing 1984.*